PROFESSIONAL PARAMEDIC

TRAUMA CARE & EMS OPERATIONS

STUDY GUIDE

VOLUME III

RICHARD BEEBE

DELMAR
CENGAGE Learning™

Australia • Brazil • Japan • Korea • Mexico • Singapore • Spain • United Kingdom • United States

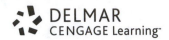

Professional Paramedic:
   Trauma Care & EMS Operations
   Study Guide
Richard Beebe

Vice President, Career and Professional
   Editorial: Dave Garza

Director of Learning Solutions: Sandy Clark

Senior Acquisitions Editor: Janet Maker

Managing Editor: Larry Main

Senior Product Manager: Jennifer A. Starr

Editorial Assistant: Amy Wetsel

Vice President, Career and Professional
   Marketing: Jennifer Baker

Marketing Director: Deborah S. Yarnell

Senior Marketing Manager: Erin Coffin

Associate Marketing Manager: Shanna Gibbs

Production Director: Wendy Troeger

Production Manager: Mark Bernard

Senior Content Project Manager:
   Jennifer Hanley

Art Director: Benjamin Gleeksman

ISBN-13: 978-1-4283-2349-0
ISBN-10: 1-4283-2349-X

Delmar

5 Maxwell Drive

Clifton Park, NY 12065-2919

USA

Cengage Learning is a leading provider of customized learning solutions with office locations around the globe, including Singapore, the United Kingdom, Australia, Mexico, Brazil, and Japan. Locate your local office at: **international.cengage.com/region**

Cengage Learning products are represented in Canada by Nelson Education, Ltd.

To learn more about Delmar, visit **www.cengage.com/delmar**

Purchase any of our products at your local college store or at our preferred online store **www.cengagebrain.com**

NOTICE TO THE READER

Publisher does not warrant or guarantee any of the products described herein or perform any independent analysis in connection with any of the product information contained herein. Publisher does not assume, and expressly disclaims, any obligation to obtain and include information other than that provided to it by the manufacturer. The reader is expressly warned to consider and adopt all safety precautions that might be indicated by the activities described herein and to avoid all potential hazards. By following the instructions contained herein, the reader willingly assumes all risks in connection with such instructions. The publisher makes no representations or warranties of any kind, including but not limited to, the warranties of fitness for particular purpose or merchantability, nor are any such representations implied with respect to the material set forth herein, and the publisher takes no responsibility with respect to such material. The publisher shall not be liable for any special, consequential, or exemplary damages resulting, in whole or part, from the readers' use of, or reliance upon, this material.

Printed in the United States of America
1 2 3 4 5 6 7 15 14 13 12 11

CONTENTS

PREFACE

We are pleased to offer a *Study Guide* to accompany *Professional Paramedic Volume III: Trauma Care and EMS Operations*. Inside these pages you will find tools to help you practice and prepare for success in your paramedic program, on the certification exam, and beyond.

Features

This Study Guide contains the following features:

Section I: Case Studies & Practice Questions

Divided by chapters, these features review the terms and concepts that are discussed in the corresponding chapter in the book.

- *Case Studies* present a new scenario intended to reinforce content contained within each chapter. Like the case studies in the textbook, each of the cases include critical thinking questions that prompt you to test your knowledge of the concepts presented in the case, and likewise the corresponding chapters. These activities help you develop and fine-tune the decision-making skills that ultimately relate to your success in treating patients.
- *25 Practice Questions* per chapter allow you to practice your knowledge of the content presented in the textbook. Questions include a variety of styles— multiple choice, short answer, and fill-in-the blank —to ensure that you master the content.

Section II: NREMT Skills for Paramedic Certification

This section contains the Paramedic skills that you will be tested on as part of the National Registry exam. You will want to practice the steps in the skills and ensure that you are confident in a successful completion of each skill prior to the exam.

Visit **www.nremt.org** for up-to-date information on the National Registry and certification exams.

Section III: Answers to Questions

The answers to the questions provided in this Study Guide offer you an opportunity to evaluate your knowledge of the terms and concepts presented in *Professional Paramedic Volume III: Trauma Care and EMS Operations*.

About the Technical Writer/Series Co-Authors

Richard Beebe MS, BSN, NREMT-P

Richard Beebe has served in Fire/EMS, commercial EMS, volunteer EMS and as a municipal Paramedic. During that time he has served as a volunteer crew chief, a squad Captain, and Paramedic Supervisor. Currently Mr. Beebe continues to serve as a civilian Paramedic for the Guilderland Police Department, outside of Albany, New York.

Dr. Jeff Myers, DO, EdM, NREMT-P, FAAEM

Dr. Myers is board certified in Emergency Medicine. Dr. Myers is currently on faculty at the State University of New York, University at Buffalo; and serves as the Associate System EMS Medical Director and EMS Fellowship Director at the Erie County Medical Center, where he is an active member of the physician response team. He recently became the medical director for the Paramedic program at the Erie Community College and also holds the position of the Director of the Behling Simulation Center at the University at Buffalo, an interprofessional simulation center that brings together learners from all health professions.

Also Available

- *Professional Paramedic Volume I: Foundations of Paramedic Care/Order#: 978-1-4283-2345-2*
- *Study Guide to accompany Professional Paramedic Volume I: Foundations of Paramedic Care/Order#: 978-1-4283-2346-9*
- *Professional Paramedic Volume II: Medical Emergencies, Maternal Health & Pediatrics Order#: 978-1-4283-2351-3*
- *Study Guide to accompany Professional Paramedic Volume II: Medical Emergencies, Maternal Health & Pediatrics/ Order#: 978-1-4283-2352-0*

Please visit us online for more learning tools for this series, available on our *Online Companion* site, as well as to view other EMS titles: **www.cengage.com/community/ems**

ACING THE CERTIFICATION EXAM: AN INTRODUCTION TO TEST-TAKING STRATEGIES

Introduction

Test time. Whether you are preparing for a certification test or a hiring test, the thought of an examination strikes fear in many people's hearts. The fear is so common that psychologists even have a diagnosis called test anxiety. However, testing does not have to be that way. Evaluations are simply an instrument to determine if you were effectively taught the information intended, or if you have the knowledge base necessary to do the job. That's all! If the purpose of testing is so simple, then why do so many people become so anxious when test time comes? Several factors play into test anxiety and why so many people have such fears of testing. However, these can be overcome. With the assistance of this guide, you too can be better prepared and calmer on examination day.

Test Obstacles

Test obstacles are issues that complicate test taking. If we view test taking as simply an avenue to determine the individual's comprehension of the material, then test obstacles are barriers to the process. There are many issues that may create test obstacles. We will discuss a few.

Mental

Mental test obstacles can sometimes be the greatest hurdles to overcome. Mental preparation for a test can be as important as intellectual preparation. So often, many people have failed an exam before they even begin. Issues that arise out of mental obstacles are:

- feeling unprepared
- feeling incompetent
- fear of taking tests
- fear of failure

Overcoming these obstacles can be your greatest asset when testing. Not allowing yourself to be beaten before entering the testing area can make the difference between success and failure on the exam.

Physical

Improper rest, poor eating habits, and lack of exercise can be some of the physical obstacles to overcome. When preparing for tests, always ensure that you get plenty of rest the night before, have a well-balanced meal before the test, and ensure you have a regiment of proper exercise. Physical obstacles are typically the easiest to overcome; however, they are the most overlooked.

Emotional

The emotional obstacles are often the most vague with which to deal. Much like mental obstacles, emotional obstacles can cause a person to do poorly on an exam well before they enter the room. Stress related issues that can interfere with test taking are:

- family concerns
- work-related concerns
- financial concerns

Emotional issues can cause a person to lose focus, cloud decision-making skills, and become distracted. Overcoming these obstacles requires a conscious effort to ensure that emotions do not interfere with the test.

Preparing to Take a Test

Before the Test

1. Start preparing for the examination. For certification exams, start the first day of class. You can do this by reading your syllabus carefully to find out when your exams will be, how many there will be, and how much they are weighed into your grade.
2. For certification classes, plan reviews as part of your regular weekly study schedule; a significant amount of time should be used to review the entire material for the class.
3. Reviews are much more than reading and reviewing class assignments. You need to read over your class notes and ask yourself questions on the material you don't know well. (If your notes are relatively complete and well organized, you may find that very little rereading of the textbook for detail is needed.) You may want to create a study group for these reviews to reinforce your learning.
4. Review for several short periods rather than one long period. You will find that you are able to retain information better and get less fatigued.
5. Turn the main points of each topic or heading into questions and check to see if the answers come to you quickly and correctly. Do not try to guess the types of questions; instead, concentrate on understanding the material.

During the Test

1. Preview the test before you answer anything. This gets you thinking about the material. Make sure to note the point value of each question. This will give you some ideas on how best to allocate your time.
2. Quickly calculate how much time you should allow for each question. A general rule of thumb is that you should be able to answer 50 questions per hour. This averages out to one question every 1.2 seconds. However, make sure you clearly understand the amount of time you have to complete the test.
3. Read the directions CAREFULLY. (Can more than one answer be correct? Are you penalized for guessing?) Never assume that you know what the directions say.
4. Answer the easy questions first. This will give you confidence and a feel for the flow of the test. Only answer the ones for which you are sure of the correct answer.
5. Go back to the difficult questions. The questions you have answered so far may provide some indication of the answers.
6. Answer all questions (unless you are penalized for wrong answers).
7. Generally, once the test begins, the proctor can ONLY reread the question. He/she cannot provide any further information.
8. Circle key words in difficult questions. This will force you to focus on the central point.
9. Narrow your options on the question to two answers. Many times, a question will be worded with two answers that are obviously inaccurate, and two answers that are close. However, only one is correct. If you can narrow your options to two, guessing may be easier. For example, if you have four options on a question, then you have a 25% chance of getting the question correct when guessing. If you can narrow the options to two answers, then you increase to a 50% chance of selecting the correct choice.
10. Use all of the time allotted for the test. If you have extra time, review your answers for accuracy. However, be careful of making changes on questions of which you are not sure. People often change the answers to questions of which they were not sure, when their first guess was correct.

After the Test

Relax. The test has been turned in. You can spend hours second-guessing what you could have done, but the test is complete. For certification tests, follow up to see if you can find out what objectives you did well and what areas you could improve. Review your test if you can; otherwise, try to remap the areas of question and refocus your studying.

Summary

Test taking does not have to be overwhelming. The obstacles to testing can be overcome and conquered through solid strategies and preparation. Initiating an effective plan, following it, and mentally preparing for a test can be your greatest tools to test success.

Acing the Certification Exam: An Introduction to Test-Taking Strategies

CASE STUDIES & PRACTICE QUESTIONS

CHAPTER 1

TRAUMA OVERVIEW

Case Study

The squeal of wheels came just moments before the sickening thud of metal on metal. Deadman's Curve had claimed another. The sharp turn in the country road did not have the modern safety features that highway engineering had created for modern roadways to reduce vehicular trauma, such as a guardrail or banked curves.

A farmer quickly runs to the corner. Sure enough, there is a pair of fresh skid marks overlying old skid marks and a distinct trail of broken underbrush that leads to the car resting against the tree.

Looking through the brush, the farmer can see an older model sedan with its front windshield popped out. He looks into the front seat, but no one is there. He then hears a low moaning under the bushes.

Critical Thinking Questions

1. What are the predictable injuries based on the mechanism of injury?

   _____

   _____

2. What modern safety equipment might have prevented these injuries?

   _____

   _____

The driver is conscious, but just barely. The farmer can see a shiny reflection that he figures must be the man's skull under the scalp laceration. He notices copious bleeding from the scalp wound, but he assumes the hidden head injury underlying the wound is probably a more life-threatening condition.

The farmer moves to the driver's head to hold manual stabilization of the neck. When the farmer looks up, he can see his wife on the shoulder of the road calling 9-1-1 from her cell phone. Using the GPS application she downloaded to her phone, she gives the county fire dispatcher the exact coordinates of the sedan.

Critical Thinking Questions

3. What is the most appropriate triage decision here?

   _____

   _____

4. Does this patient meet major trauma criteria?

   _____

   _____

Practice Questions

Multiple Choice

Select the best answer for each of the following questions.

1. What causes liquefaction necrosis?
   a. mechanical force
   b. electricity
   c. chemicals
   d. radiation

2. What is the best way to reduce trauma deaths?
   a. injury prevention programs
   b. rapid first response
   c. advanced life support
   d. trauma center systems

3. DWI laws are examples of what method of injury prevention?
   a. education
   b. eradication
   c. enforcement
   d. engineering

4. What is the name of the pivotal paper that started the trauma care movement?
   a. Death in the Ditch
   b. Accidental Death and Disability
   c. Death and Trauma
   d. Trauma Care

5. What level of trauma center requires in-house trauma surgeons to be on staff?
   a. Level I Trauma Center
   b. Level II Trauma Center
   c. Level III Trauma Center
   d. Level IV Trauma Center

6. Who is credited with creating triage?
   a. General Letterman
   b. Baron Dominique Jean Larrey
   c. American College of Surgeons
   d. Federal Centers for Disease Control

7. When organs inside the body, like the heart, strike the sternum during a motor vehicle collision, this is an example of which of Newton's laws of motion?
   a. first law of motion
   b. second law of motion
   c. third law of motion
   d. fourth law of motion

8. Injuries to the patient's knees, and an imprint of the knees on the crash bar below the steering wheel, indicate which patient pathway of travel?
   a. down-and-under pathway
   b. forward pathway
   c. up-and-over pathway
   d. none of the above

9. What is the most catastrophic mechanism in a motor vehicle collision?
   a. ejection
   b. rollover
   c. rotational
   d. front impact

10. A hollow nose bullet increases trauma through what characteristic?
    a. deformity
    b. size
    c. tumbling
    d. yaw

11. Ruptured eardrums occur as a _____ blast injury.
    a. primary
    b. secondary
    c. tertiary
    d. quaternary

12. Trauma patients with which of the following conditions should NOT be transported immediately to a trauma center?
    a. fall of 20 feet
    b. hypotension
    c. pregnant
    d. two proximal long-bone fractures

13. A driver locks out his arms on the steering wheel prior to a collision. Which of the following are predictable injuries?
    a. wrist injuries
    b. shoulder injuries
    c. cervical injuries
    d. all of the above

14. Isolated injury to the left shoulder and ribs is most likely in which type of collision?
    a. rollover
    b. frontal impact
    c. lateral impact
    d. rear-end impact

15. Which of the following is part of the occupant restraint system?
    a. seat belt
    b. head rests
    c. airbags
    d. all of the above

Short Answer

Write a brief answer to each of the following questions.

16. List three similarities between trauma and infectious disease.

    _____

    _____

17. Define triage.

    _____

    _____

18. Differentiate overtriage and undertriage.

_____

_____

19. What is the advantage of identifying the mechanism of injury?

_____

_____

20. Differentiate stab wounds inflicted by women from those inflicted by men.

_____

_____

Fill in the Blank

Complete each sentence by adding the appropriate word in the provided blanks.

21. Trauma is defined as injury caused by _____ _____.

22. When a projectile breaks the skin, it is called a _____ _____.

23. In kinetic energy, the _____ is more important than the _____.

24. Motorcyclists try to _____ _____ the bike to prevent injury.

25. Protection from projectiles is provided by _____ _____ _____.

CHAPTER 2

TRAUMATIC BRAIN INJURY

Case Study

Chief Concern

On a dark and rainy night, the scene is ablaze with flashing lights created by the half dozen emergency vehicles present. Traffic in the intersection is tied in a knot. Police are carefully weaving cars through the snarled traffic, trying not to endanger rescuers as they clear the scene for more emergency vehicles.

One vehicle has T-boned another vehicle and pushed it up against the signal light pole. Fire rescue is busy extricating the patient from the first vehicle. Meanwhile, the first ambulance on scene is already preparing the driver from the second vehicle for transport to the trauma center. EMS command directs Mohamed and his partner, Nikhil, to assist the first vehicle.

Critical Thinking Questions

1. What are some of the possible traumatic brain injuries that would be suspected based on the mechanism of injury?

   _____

   _____

2. Are any of these traumatic brain injuries potentially life-threatening conditions?

   _____

   _____

History

The pinned driver is visibly conscious and sitting upright in the car. Struck in the driver's side, with over 18 inches of intrusion into the driver's compartment, this crash meets the major trauma criteria for transportation to the trauma center. Unfortunately, since the rainy weather precludes the helicopter from flying, the patient will be going to the trauma center "by ground."

Standing outside of the action circle, Nikhil communicates with the firefighter inside the car who is holding head stabilization while rescue is prying the doors. It seems that the patient has taken out the driver's side window with his head and is bleeding profusely from the left temple. He also complains of severe headache. As for the accident, he has a vague memory of sliding through the intersection but remembers little else.

At that moment, the rescue captain taps Nikhil on the shoulder and points to the sidewalk. "That lady says he was knocked out. May have been unconscious for as much as two or three minutes." Looking toward the sidewalk, Nikhil sees an apprehensive middle-aged woman. "Mohamed," Nikhil asks, "could you please interview her about the accident?"

Critical Thinking Questions

1. What is the most important element of the history for a trauma patient?

   _____

   _____

2. What *specific* elements of the history should the Paramedic obtain from this patient?

_____

_____

Examination

The firefighters rapidly extricate the patient to a long backboard. One firefighter is holding both manual stabilization of the cervical spine as well as a 4 × 4 dressing over the laceration to the patient's left-side midline, just above the temple.

While the firefighters proceed to strap the patient to the backboard, and before the head blocks are put in place, Nikhil lifts the dressing and sees a jagged three-inch laceration underneath. Of greater concern is the appearance of a "step off," an even surface over the temple. Replacing the dressing, Nikhil speaks to the firefighter. "I don't think we should use head blocks. Just keep manual stabilization and be careful where you press. I think he might have an open skull fracture." The firefighter nods in acknowledgment, waving off the head blocks and calling out to his lieutenant, "I think I am going in on this one."

Critical Thinking Questions

1. What are the elements of the physical examination of a patient with suspected herniation syndrome?

_____

_____

2. Why are vital signs a critical element in this examination?

_____

_____

Assessment

"Do you remember what happened?" asks Nikhil. The patient has a vague memory of the events. According to the report, he slid through the intersection, against the red light, and may have been unconscious. However, Mohamed is not convinced that the woman is a reliable reporter.

Based on the questionable history and the high energy involved in the crash, Nikhil assumes that the potential exists for a head injury. And understanding that head injury is the number one killer of trauma victims, he decides to make this patient a high priority patient.

Critical Thinking Questions

1. What is the significance of the area impacted?

_____

_____

2. What is the patient's prognosis?

_____

_____

Treatment

While en route to the trauma center, Nikhil ensures the patient's airway is patent while reassuring the patient that everything that can be done for him is being done. Nikhil checks the patient's blood sugar while obtaining venous access and is satisfied with the result of 120 mg/dL. Readjusting the oxygen mask, Nikhil proceeds with a head-to-toe assessment.

Critical Thinking Questions

1. What is the national standard of care of patients with suspected traumatic brain injury?

_____

_____

2. What are some of the patient-specific concerns and considerations that the Paramedic should consider when applying this plan of care that is intended to treat a broad patient population presenting with acute herniation syndrome?

_____

_____

Evaluation

Suddenly, the patient becomes uncooperative and combative. He keeps asking, "Where am I? Where am I?" indicating short-term memory loss.

The patient then seizes and becomes unresponsive. Calling out the patient's name to no avail, Nikhil executes a sternal rub. The patient postures. Nikhil then starts to hyperventilate the patient.

Critical Thinking Questions

1. What are some of the predictable complications associated with acute herniation syndrome?

_____

_____

2. What are some of the predictable complications associated with the treatment of acute herniation syndrome?

_____

_____

Disposition

Wheeling the patient into the emergency department, Mohamed and Nikhil are met by the neurosurgeon. Penlight in hand, he checks the patient's pupils as he hears the story. "Let's prepare for intubation, and can I get some sedation for the patient as well?" he calls out.

In the blink of an eye, the patient who has occupied the crew's entire attention is taken away. Nikhil sighs.

Critical Thinking Questions

1. What is the most appropriate transport decision that will get the patient to definitive care?

_____

_____

2. What are the advantages of transporting a patient with suspected acute herniation syndrome to these hospitals, even if that means bypassing other hospitals in the process?

_____

_____

Practice Questions
Multiple Choice

Select the best answer for each of the following questions.

1. What is the leading cause of traumatic brain injury?
   a. assault
   b. falls
   c. gunshot wounds
   d. motor vehicle collisions

2. The peak incidence of traumatic brain injury occurs with people who are _____ years of age.
   a. 15 to 24
   b. 24 to 30
   c. 30 to 50
   d. >55

3. Which of the following is NOT considered an extracerebral hemorrhage?
   a. subarachnoid
   b. concussion
   c. subdural
   d. epidural

4. Which brain injury is likely to occur in a coup–contrecoup injury?
   a. cerebral concussion
   b. cerebral contusion
   c. cerebral hemorrhage
   d. cerebral anoxia

5. Which of the following is least likely to form a hematoma and become a space-occupying lesion that leads to herniation?
   a. subarachnoid hemorrhage
   b. subdural hematoma
   c. epidural hematoma
   d. cerebral laceration

6. What is the most likely traumatic brain injury in shaken baby syndrome?
   a. subarachnoid hemorrhage
   b. subdural hematoma
   c. epidural hematoma
   d. cerebral laceration

7. Which traumatic brain injury has the lowest incidence, yet has the highest mortality?
   a. subarachnoid hemorrhage
   b. subdural hematoma
   c. epidural hematoma
   d. cerebral laceration

8. Which of the following is NOT a supratentorial herniation?
   a. central herniation
   b. uncal herniation
   c. tonsillar herniation
   d. cingulate herniation

9. Which herniation causes compression of the cerebellum?
   a. central herniation
   b. uncal herniation
   c. tonsillar herniation
   d. cingulate herniation

10. Which herniation can mimic a cervical spine injury?
    a. central herniation
    b. uncal herniation
    c. tonsillar herniation
    d. cingulate herniation

11. Patients with _____ herniation may present with confusion, loss of short-term memory, and even combativeness.
    a. central
    b. uncal
    c. tonsillar
    d. cingulate

12. Triple flexion (hip, knees, and ankles) can be seen in which condition?
    a. decorticate rigidity
    b. extensor posturing
    c. decerebrate rigidity
    d. none of the above

13. What is the first change in respiration as a result of increased intracranial pressure?
    a. Cheyne–Stokes respiration
    b. central neurogenic hyperventilation
    c. apneustic breathing
    d. agonal respirations

14. "Breath-holding" phenomenon is seen with which of the following conditions?
    a. Cheyne–Stokes respiration
    b. central neurogenic hyperventilation
    c. apneustic breathing
    d. agonal respirations

15. An agitated and confused patient is what level on the modified Rancho Los Amigos scale?
    a. X
    b. VI
    c. IV
    d. II

Short Answer

Write a brief answer to each of the following questions.

16. Define traumatic brain injury.

_____

_____

17. What is the symptom pattern associated with a concussion?

_____

_____

18. What is the Monroe–Kellie hypothesis?

_____

_____

19. What is "hippus"?

_____

_____

20. Name three signs of a basilar skull fracture.

_____

_____

Fill in the Blank

Complete each sentence by adding the appropriate word in the provided blanks.

21. Shifting of the brain due to an accumulation of blood is called the _____ _____.

22. An acute subdural hematoma occurs in less than _____ to _____ hours.

23. The _____ _____ helps to differentiate a subdural hematoma from an epidural hematoma.

24. The formula for cerebral perfusion pressure is _____ _____ _____ (_____) minus _____ _____ (_____).

25. A premorbid breathing pattern is ataxic or _____ breathing.

CHAPTER 3

NECK AND FACIAL TRAUMA

Case Study

Chief Concern

"Ah, Dr. Le Fort," Megan sighs as she approaches the patient. "I hope you taught me well." The ceiling overhead at the fire scene had collapsed onto the firefighters performing overhaul below. One of the wooden structural beams struck a firefighter across the face. The firefighter wasn't wearing his helmet, all but assuring he will be facing recriminations in the future. At this moment, however, Megan's concern is the firefighter's obvious facial lacerations.

Critical Thinking Questions

1. What are some of the possible facial injuries that would be suspected based on the mechanism of injury?

   _____

   _____

2. Are any of these facial injuries potentially life-threatening conditions?

   _____

   _____

History

After completing her primary assessment, Megan proceeds with getting a little patient history. Apparently there was a loud crack and suddenly the whole ceiling caved in. After the dust settled, fellow firefighters found the patient under the rubble. While trying to maintain his head in neutral alignment, the firefighters carefully removed the debris while the lieutenant radioed for EMS.

Critical Thinking Questions

1. What are the important elements of the history that the Paramedic should obtain?

   _____

   _____

2. What additional elements of the history should the Paramedic obtain?

   _____

   _____

Examination

The large amount of blood coming from the patient's face is quite distracting. Through the blood, Megan sees the faint outline of a wooden crossbeam on the patient's face. Focusing on the task at hand, Megan methodically assesses the patient while her partner maintains continuous manual stabilization of the cervical spine.

Critical Thinking Questions

1. What are the elements of the physical examination of a patient with suspected Le Fort fractures?

_____

_____

2. Why would a cranial nerve exam be a critical element in this examination?

_____

_____

Assessment

The patient suddenly becomes agitated and starts to try to remove his immobilization, yelling, "I can't see! I can't see!" Speaking calmly into his ear, Megan says, "Calm down and let me check your eyes." Grabbing a penlight, she inspects the patient's eyes. His pupils still seem reactive and she does not see any black spots, which are suggestive of a ruptured globe. "What do you see?" she asks. "It was like someone drew a curtain over my left eye," he replies.

Critical Thinking Questions

1. What is the significance of the patient's loss of vision?

_____

_____

2. What is the patient's prognosis?

_____

_____

Treatment

Lying the patient down onto a backboard seems self-defeating, since his airway will simply fill up with blood, creating another problem. Megan elects to apply a cervical collar and a short-board device to help maintain neutral cervical alignment while allowing the patient to sit upright on the stretcher. In that position, the blood might drain naturally and not become as much of an issue.

Critical Thinking Questions

1. What is the first priority in the care of patients with suspected midface fractures?

_____

_____

2. What is the next priority in the care of patients with suspected midface fractures?

_____

_____

Evaluation

Blood is pouring out of the patient's nose and the Paramedic's efforts to stem the flow are not working. Almost on cue, the patient announces he is "lightheaded" as the EMT announces his blood pressure is 90 on 50. Megan faces a tough decision. When the patient sits up, he has an airway and no blood pressure. When the patient lies flat, he has a blood pressure but no airway.

Critical Thinking Questions

1. What are some of the predictable complications associated with midface fractures?

   _____

   _____

2. What are some of the predictable complications associated with the treatments for midface fractures?

   _____

   _____

Disposition

With the patient in the left lateral recumbent position, Megan gives report to the trauma center. The litany of injuries is lengthy and the loud siren only serves to emphasize the life-threatening nature of the trauma. The trauma nurse receiving report signs off with, "See you in Trauma Bay One."

Critical Thinking Questions

1. What is the most appropriate transport decision that will get the patient to definitive care?

   _____

   _____

2. What are the advantages of transporting a patient with suspected midface fractures to these hospitals, even if that means bypassing other hospitals in the process?

   _____

   _____

Practice Questions
Multiple Choice

Select the best answer for each of the following questions.

1. Which of the following terms describes a horizontal fracture of the maxilla?
   a. Le Fort type I
   b. Le Fort type II
   c. Le Fort type III
   d. Le Fort type IV

2. Craniofacial dysfunction was originally referred to by what name?
   a. Le Fort type I
   b. Le Fort type II
   c. Le Fort type III
   d. Le Fort type IV

3. What is the largest risk in an orbital fracture?
   a. damage to the infraorbital nerve
   b. entrapment of extraocular nerves
   c. rupture of the medial rectus muscle
   d. retinal nerve detachment

4. What does a red spot in the dentin suggest?
   a. Ellis I tooth fracture
   b. Ellis II tooth fracture
   c. Ellis III tooth fracture
   d. Ellis IV tooth fracture

5. What is the most "sight-threatening" injury to the eye?
   a. traumatic iritis
   b. subconjunctival hemorrhage
   c. hyphema
   d. corneal abrasion

6. Which of the following is found in Zone I of a neck injury?
   a. jugular vein
   b. cranial nerves
   c. lung apices
   d. pharynx

7. Which of the following is found in Zone II of a neck injury?
   a. subclavian artery
   b. cranial nerves
   c. lung apices
   d. pharynx

8. If the patient has trouble looking upward, the _____ is most likely entrapped.
   a. inferior rectus
   b. extraocular nerve
   c. medial rectus
   d. infraorbital nerve

9. If the patient has trouble looking laterally, the _____ is most likely entrapped.
   a. inferior rectus
   b. extraocular nerve
   c. medial rectus
   d. infraorbital nerve

10. Severe eye pain and a small black spot in the sclera would suggest what condition to the Paramedic?
    a. traumatic iritis
    b. subconjunctival hemorrhage
    c. hyphema
    d. globe rupture

11. Which of the following conditions is most benign?
    a. traumatic iritis
    b. subconjunctival hemorrhage
    c. hyphema
    d. corneal abrasion

12. Which of the following neck injuries is likely to present like a stroke?
    a. blunt injury with hematoma to the carotids
    b. dissection of the external jugular veins
    c. thyroid injury
    d. carotid artery dissection

13. Which of the following is suggestive of a rapidly expanding hematoma in the throat?
    a. hoarseness of voice
    b. neck swelling
    c. difficulty swallowing
    d. all of the above

14. Which type of eyelid lacerations will likely be treated by an ophthalmologist?
    a. inferior
    b. lateral
    c. medial
    d. superior

15. Which of the following symptoms will be seen with a tympanic membrane perforation?
    a. severe vertigo
    b. nausea
    c. hearing loss
    d. all of the above

Short Answer

Write a brief answer to each of the following questions.

16. What are the two mechanisms suspected of causing orbital blowout fractures?

    _____

    _____

17. Why do mandibular fractures usually occur in pairs?

    _____

    _____

18. If the patient's voice suddenly becomes hoarse, what should the Paramedic suspect?

    _____

    _____

19. What are the three zones of neck injuries?

    _____

    _____

20. Describe the paper bag effect.

    _____

    _____

Fill in the Blank

Complete each sentence by adding the appropriate word in the provided blanks.

21. The Paramedic who sees blood in the ear (i.e., ottorrhea) following an explosion should suspect _____ _____ _____.

22. A _____ _____ can lead to cauliflower ear, which often occurs in professional fighters.

23. Unilateral nonreactive pupils can occur with _____ _____.

24. Tears in the retina that cause vitreous fluid in the globe to leak behind the retina can lead to _____ _____.

25. The famous classical anatomist who classified facial fractures was _____ _____ _____.

CHAPTER 4

SPINAL TRAUMA

Case Study

Chief Concern

The scene is like something from a gang-related musical. One group lines one wall of the alley, whereas another group takes a position near the other wall. Two lone combatants square off in the middle of the alley until the distant wail of a siren permeates the night air. Everyone scatters for cover, but not before one assailant manages to stab his fleeing rival in the back.

When EMS arrives, the patient is prone in the alley, with the knife visible in the middle of his back. Another crowd, this time made up of curious onlookers, gathers as police start establishing a perimeter.

Critical Thinking Questions

1. What are some of the possible medical causes of paralysis?

_____

_____

2. What are some of the possible traumatic causes of paralysis?

_____

_____

History

Except for the knife wound, the patient is a healthy young male who has no significant past medical history. The Paramedic hears murmurs of "Something like this can cut down a young man in the prime of his life" from the crowd. However, his focus is on the patient. The Paramedic remembers that trauma is the number one killer of this patient population.

Critical Thinking Questions

1. What is the first element of the history that a Paramedic should obtain?

_____

_____

2. What other elements of the history should the Paramedic try to obtain?

_____

_____

Examination

"Curious," the Paramedic states out loud. "Only one-half of his body is paralyzed." Although the patient has a peculiar presentation, the Paramedic's partner reminds him that the aorta lies on the other side of the spinal column and that when a knife lacerates the spine it may also pierce the aorta.

That last statement increases the situation's urgency. On one side, the Paramedics know that they have to handle the patient carefully to prevent further injury. On the other hand, internal hemorrhage can potentially be a life-threatening condition, one only a trauma surgeon can correct.

Critical Thinking Questions

1. What are the elements of the physical examination of a patient with suspected spinal cord syndrome?

_____

_____

2. Why is a dermatome-focused neurological examination a critical element in this examination?

_____

_____

Assessment

The Paramedic reassures the patient that everything that can be done for him is being done. This statement does not seem to comfort the young man. Having told the Paramedic that he's a recent new dad, he clearly understands the implications of paralysis, no matter the degree of disability.

Critical Thinking Questions

1. What is the significance of the loss of feeling on one side of the body and loss of movement on the other side?

_____

_____

2. What diagnosis did the Paramedic announce to the patient?

_____

_____

Treatment

Electing to keep the patient supine, the Paramedics use a "scoop" stretcher that operates like a pair of clamshells to scoop the patient up and place him on the backboard. The board is already padded so his chest and head will be parallel.

With the patient "packaged," the Paramedics proceed toward the ambulance. A young police officer tags along, asking if the Paramedics can pull the knife and leave it as evidence. Before the Paramedics can turn to answer, a police sergeant intervenes with the stern words, "Leave it be."

Critical Thinking Questions

1. What is the national standard of care of patients with suspected spinal cord injury?

_____

_____

2. What are some of the patient-specific concerns and considerations that the Paramedic should consider when applying this plan of care that is intended to treat a broad patient population presenting with spinal cord injury?

_____

_____

Evaluation

While en route to the hospital, the patient has a sudden loss of bladder control. "Time to repeat the primary," declares the Paramedic. Concerned the incontinence might forebode future neurogenic shock, the Paramedic wants to have a firm handle on the patient's hemodynamic status.

Critical Thinking Questions

1. Why were these spinal cord injury complications predictable?

   _____

   _____

2. What potentially life-threatening complication could occur because of spinal cord injury?

   _____

   _____

Disposition

Despite the potentially devastating injury, the patient remains stable throughout the transport and is delivered to the trauma center in stable condition. Transferred to the care of the trauma team in Trauma Bay Two, the crew goes back into service as the trauma team wonders how they are going to care for the prone patient.

Critical Thinking Questions

1. What is the most appropriate transport decision that will get the patient to definitive care?

   _____

   _____

2. What are the advantages of transporting a patient with suspected spinal cord injury to these hospitals, even if that means bypassing other hospitals in the process?

   _____

   _____

Practice Questions

Multiple Choice

Select the best answer for each of the following questions.

1. Which term means a complete disruption of the spinal cord?
   a. spinal transection
   b. spinal dislocation
   c. spinal subluxation
   d. spinal herniation

2. Which syndrome is described by loss of motor function but retention of touch and position sense?
   a. anterior cord syndrome
   b. Brown–Sequard syndrome
   c. central cord syndrome
   d. posterior cord syndrome

3. Which syndrome is described by hemiplegia on one side and hemiparesis on the other?
   a. anterior cord syndrome
   b. Brown–Sequard syndrome
   c. central cord syndrome
   d. posterior cord syndrome

4. Which syndrome is described by motor weakness in the upper extremities?
   a. anterior cord syndrome
   b. Brown–Sequard syndrome
   c. central cord syndrome
   d. posterior cord syndrome

5. Which of the following is NOT considered a "high risk" mechanism for spinal cord injury?
   a. fall of greater than two stories (adult)
   b. gunshot to the abdomen
   c. ejection during a motor vehicle collision
   d. death of another occupant in a motor vehicle collision

6. Abnormal flexion does NOT occur in which of the following situations?
   a. headfirst falls
   b. assault with a baseball bat from the rear
   c. sudden deceleration motor vehicle collision
   d. suicide by hanging

7. A glancing blow to the chin, such as by a fist, would cause injury by which process?
   a. rotation
   b. flexion
   c. extension
   d. compression

8. A judicial hanging causes death by which process?
   a. rotation
   b. distraction
   c. extension
   d. flexion

9. A diving accident, such as diving headfirst into shallow water and striking bottom, would most likely cause spinal cord injury by which process?
   a. compression
   b. distraction
   c. extension
   d. rotation

10. Which of the following decreases an examination's reliability?
    a. acute stress reaction
    b. painful distracting injury
    c. language barrier
    d. all of the above

11. While testing for strength during an examination for neurological compromise, an inability to lift a limb would be _____ on the grading scale.
    a. 0
    b. 1
    c. 2
    d. 3

12. An inability to abduct the fingers suggests injury at which location?
    a. C5
    b. C6
    c. C7
    d. C8

13. Numbness at the lateral side of the antecubital fossa suggests spinal cord injury at which level?
    a. C1 to C3
    b. C3 to C5
    c. C5 to C7
    d. C7 to T1

14. What is the optimal method of moving a patient to a backboard?
    a. log roll
    b. four-person lift
    c. split rigid stretcher
    d. long axis drag

15. Which symptom is NOT consistent with the triad of symptoms seen in neurogenic shock?
    a. tachycardia
    b. bradycardia
    c. hypotension
    d. vasodilation

Short Answer

Write a brief answer to each of the following questions.

16. Which syndrome is due to a "deadman's fall"?

    _____

    _____

17. Why are patients with Down syndrome more prone to potentially life-threatening cervical spine injury?

    _____

    _____

18. What is sacral sparing?

    _____

    _____

19. Describe the performance and implications of a Babinski test.

    _____

    _____

20. What is selective spinal immobilization?

    _____

    _____

Fill in the Blank

Complete each sentence by adding the appropriate word in the provided blanks.

21. The former name for tetraplegia was _____.

22. The ascending nerve tracts are _____ tracts called the _____ tracts, whereas the descending nerve tracts are _____ tracts called the _____ tracts.

23. Loss of bowel/bladder control is seen in sacral cord injury and is called _____ _____ syndrome.

24. Spinal cord injury not evident on medical imaging (CAT scan, X-ray, MRI) is called _____.

25. A painful erection is called a _____.

CHAPTER 5

THORACIC TRAUMA

Case Study
Chief Concern

"Shots fired, man down," comes the report over the radio. Mike is accompanying the SWAT team on a high-risk warrant. Though he has done dozens of these with the team, and he has trained extensively for this day, he still feels unprepared. "Was it a perp or an operative? Or maybe a civilian who innocently wandered into the line of fire during a fire fight?" he wonders as he assembles his quick-response supplies.

Critical Thinking Questions

1. What are some of the possible causes of chest trauma?

   _____

   _____

2. How is trouble breathing related to chest trauma?

   _____

   _____

History

It turns out an officer was shot through the screen door by a crazed gunman wielding a rifle as the officer attempted to serve him a warrant. The SWAT team has secured the area immediately surrounding the officer. Even though each person wants to look over his shoulder to see what is going on, each of them knows that he needs to focus on the perimeter security.

Critical Thinking Questions

1. What are the important elements of the history that a Paramedic should obtain?

   _____

   _____

2. What important medical history should also be obtained?

   _____

   _____

Examination

As Mike kneels next to the officer, he knows the officer may have an open penetrating chest trauma. However, Mike sighs in relief when he notices the officer took the round in the vest. Then he realizes the officer did not have his plate in place. Did someone already remove it? Did the officer fail to put the hard armor in place because it was hot out? In either case, it didn't really matter at that moment.

Assessment reveals that the officer has chest pain, difficulty in breathing, and an obvious contusion the size of a quarter where the bullet punched the chest under the vest. A subtle "step off" announces a rib fracture, and diminished breath sounds confirm a pneumothorax.

Critical Thinking Questions

1. What are the elements of the physical examination of a patient with chest trauma?

   _____

   _____

2. Why is auscultation a critical element in this examination?

   _____

   _____

Assessment

Mike reassures the officer that they will be moving in a few minutes. He knows the policy is to protect the patient in place until the perpetrator can be neutralized. However, he also understands the importance of rapid assessment and transport, especially for thoracic trauma.

Critical Thinking Questions

1. What is the significance of the patient's absent breath sounds?

   _____

   _____

2. Does the patient lying supine affect the Paramedic's physical findings?

   _____

   _____

Treatment

Mike watches the officer's respiratory rate climb as his pulse oximeter reading falls. He also watches the developing jugular venous distention. Reassessing the chest wall, he sees the problem. Either a bullet fragment or a second bullet has pierced the patient's skin just under the arm, in the axilla. Cursing himself for missing the wound during the primary assessment, Mike prepares to treat the sucking chest wound.

Critical Thinking Questions

1. What is the national standard of care of patients with a sucking chest wound?

   _____

   _____

2. What are alternative treatments for a sucking chest wound?

   _____

   _____

Evaluation

The officer's breathing is very shallow and his oxygen saturation has fallen below 90%. "Time to bag," Mike realizes, dreading the predictable outcome. Almost as soon as the mask hits the officer's face, Mike loses his radial pulse. Without hesitation, Mike reaches into the officer's self-aid kit and pulls out the thoracostomy needle. With a hiss of air, the radial pulse returns.

Critical Thinking Questions

1. What are some of the predictable complications associated with simple pneumothorax?

   _____

   _____

2. What are some of the predictable complications associated with the treatments for a tension pneumothorax?

   _____

   _____

Disposition

"All clear!" comes the announcement over the air. That's Mike's signal to package the patient and move out. Plenty of help is available, as the team carries their fallen comrade to the waiting medevac helicopter for the 15-minute flight to the trauma center.

Critical Thinking Questions

1. Are there any dangers associated with air medical evacuation?

   _____

   _____

2. What is the most appropriate transport decision that will get the patient to definitive care?

   _____

   _____

Practice Questions

Multiple Choice

Select the best answer for each of the following questions.

1. Which ribs protect the core organs?
   a. 1 to 3
   b. 4 to 7
   c. 8 to 10
   d. 11 to 12

2. Which of the following is NOT associated with a flail chest?
   a. rib fractures
   b. pneumothorax
   c. paradoxical motion
   d. altered mechanics of breathing

3. Air escaping the chest cavity is NOT seen in which of the following conditions?
   a. open pneumothorax
   b. sucking chest wound
   c. closed hemopneumothorax
   d. penetrating chest wound

4. Crackling lung sounds suggest which of the following conditions?
   a. sucking chest wound
   b. hemothorax
   c. pulmonary contusion
   d. simple pneumothorax

5. Which chest injury is most likely to become a life-threatening condition in the field?
   a. sucking chest wound
   b. pulmonary contusion
   c. hemopneumothorax
   d. tension pneumothorax

6. What is the most devastating thoracic vascular injury on scene?
   a. traumatic aortic disruptions
   b. myocardial contusion
   c. pericardial tamponade
   d. tension pneumothorax

7. An irregular heartbeat is suggestive of which of the following conditions?
   a. traumatic aortic disruptions
   b. myocardial contusion
   c. pericardial tamponade
   d. tension pneumothorax

8. The most common cause of diaphragmatic herniation is _____ motor vehicle collisions.
   a. frontal
   b. rear-end
   c. rollover
   d. lateral

9. As little as 150 mL of blood or fluid in the pericardium can cause which of the following conditions?
   a. tension pneumothorax
   b. diaphragmatic rupture
   c. cardiac tamponade
   d. tracheobronchial disruption

10. Subcutaneous emphysema is NOT seen in which of the following conditions?
    a. pericardial tamponade
    b. pneumothorax
    c. tracheobronchial disruption
    d. traumatic asphyxia

11. Sudden cardiac death is likely due to which of the following conditions?
    a. traumatic asphyxia
    b. commotio cordis
    c. pneumothorax
    d. tracheobronchial disruption

12. What is the preferred site for a needle decompression of a left-sided tension pneumothorax?
    a. left anterior chest, third ICS at MCL
    b. left axilla, fifth ICS at MAL
    c. right anterior chest, third ICS atMCL
    d. right axilla, fifth ICS at MAL

13. What is the least common chest injury?
    a. flail chest
    b. fractured ribs
    c. pneumothorax
    d. pulmonary contusion

14. What is the most likely cause of a pulmonary shunt?
    a. pulmonary contusion
    b. pericardial tamponade
    c. diaphragmatic rupture
    d. sucking chest wound

15. What is the least life-threatening thoracic injury?
    a. pericardial tamponade
    b. diaphragmatic rupture
    c. tension pneumothorax
    d. traumatic asphyxia

Short Answer

Write a brief answer to each of the following questions.

16. What is the important distinguishing characteristic of a flail chest?

    _____

    _____

17. What is a diaphragmatic rupture?

    _____

    _____

18. Describe the pathophysiology of commotio cordis.

    _____

    _____

19. Describe the mechanisms thought to make a pneumothorax into a tension pneumothorax.

    _____

    _____

20. Describe the difference between a simple pneumothorax and a tension pneumothorax.

    _____

    _____

Fill in the Blank

Complete each sentence by adding the appropriate word in the provided blanks.

21. The definition of a _____ _____ is two or more ribs broken in two or more places.

22. A condition in which abdominal contents are in the thoracic cavity is called _____ _____.

23. A bruise to the heart is called a _____ _____.

24. The most lethal chest trauma may be _____ _____ _____.

25. Another name for an open pneumothorax is a _____ _____ _____.

CHAPTER 6

ABDOMINAL AND GENITOURINARY TRAUMA

Case Study

Chief Concern

Although the drone of the siren is monotonous, the nature of the call is intriguing. The Paramedic intercept is flying along backcountry roads to meet up with the local volunteer fire department ambulance. The siren is not being used as much to clear traffic as it is to scare deer that might jump in front of the truck. The report is for a man kicked by a cow and complaining of abdominal pain.

Critical Thinking Questions

1. What potentially life-threatening injuries could occur from being kicked in the abdomen by a cow?

_____

_____

2. Which of these are the most life-threatening injuries?

_____

_____

History

The Paramedic arrives to find the patient being loaded onto a backboard. Ducking so as to not strike his head on the low ceiling, he is directed to a grisly looking old man who is talking a mile a minute to some young first responder who is writing down the information as fast as he can. "Yeah, I know. You would think that cows would kick backward but they can kick forward!" exclaims the farmer.

Critical Thinking Questions

1. What are the important elements of the history that a Paramedic should obtain?

_____

_____

2. Why would the use of beta blockers be problematic?

_____

_____

Examination

Lifting up the blanket, the Paramedic sees the patient's red, swollen abdomen with what appears to be a distinctive hoof print in the center. The patient insists that he does not want to be touched. However, he does allow the Paramedic to auscultate his lungs. When the Paramedic listens in the lower lobes, he slides his stethoscope over the floating ribs. The patient winces. Cutting the patient's T-shirt up to the armpit, the Paramedic can see the lower ribs on the right side are deformed.

"Vital signs are stable," announces the EMT, a kid who looks no older than 18. The Paramedic looks at the patient, who is grossly diaphoretic and ashen. All signs indicate that the patient is not stable.

Critical Thinking Questions

1. What are the elements of the physical examination of a patient with suspected internal abdominal hemorrhage?

   _____

   _____

2. Why is the fact that the patient's abdomen is distended of concern?

   _____

   _____

Assessment

The patient is loaded aboard the ambulance. It's a long drive to the local three-bed hospital, which is staffed by a physician assistant and a couple of nurses. Even though the patient's injuries are not identified on the list for major trauma in the trauma triage protocol, the mechanism of injury is cause for concern. However, air medical evacuation to a trauma center is not possible. A major weather front is encroaching on the area with thunderstorms in the forecast, and the helicopter is grounded.

Critical Thinking Questions

1. What are the potential sources of bleeding?

   _____

   _____

2. What is the Paramedic's diagnosis?

   _____

   _____

Treatment

On the way to the rural "critical access point," the Paramedic places the patient on high-flow, high-concentration oxygen and then obtains venous access. Although the Paramedic hangs a liter of fluid, he elects to keep it at the "keep vein open" (KVO) rate. After administering the fluid, the patient's pressure is holding and he is awake and alert.

"He's new," says a voice from the front compartment. The patient had apparently just moved to the farm from the city to start a new life as a hired farmhand.

Critical Thinking Questions

1. What is the national standard of care of patients with suspected abdominal injury?

   _____

   _____

2. Is there any referred pain that would be suggestive of abdominal injury?

_____

_____

Evaluation

The new monitor includes a noninvasive automatic blood pressure cuff that provides not only the systolic and diastolic pressure but also a mean arterial pressure, as well as a trend. The noninvasive blood pressure (NIBP) monitor is set to take a blood pressure every five minutes. After 30 minutes, the Paramedic prints out a trend. Clearly, the mean arterial pressure is dropping; however, it is acceptable.

Suddenly, the NIBP alarm goes off. Looking at the monitor, the Paramedic sees the pressure reads 90 systolic. The Paramedic immediately turns to the patient, who has gone unconscious.

Critical Thinking Questions

1. What are some of the predictable complications associated with an internal abdominal bleeding patient?

_____

_____

2. What are some of the predictable complications associated with the treatments for massive hemorrhage?

_____

_____

Disposition

Fortunately, although the helicopter originally could not make the scene, the front has passed and the helicopter is now waiting outside the small hospital for the patient's arrival.

The forward-thinking physician assistant called for the helicopter to stand by, in part because he knows that the helicopter has a portable machine for a FAST exam.

Critical Thinking Questions

1. What is the most appropriate transport decision that will get the patient to definitive care?

_____

_____

2. What are some of the transportation considerations?

_____

_____

Practice Questions
Multiple Choice

Select the best answer for each of the following questions.

1. Which of the following organs is NOT prone to subcapsular hematomas?
   a. kidneys
   b. liver
   c. intestines
   d. spleen

2. Which of the following will NOT refer pain to the back?
   a. liver
   b. pancreas
   c. kidneys
   d. aorta

3. The ligamentum teres is likely to injure which of the following organs?
   a. liver
   b. kidneys
   c. spleen
   d. pancreas

4. Bruising of the left flank is most likely due to bleeding from which of the following organs?
   a. liver
   b. kidneys
   c. spleen
   d. pancreas

5. Which portion of the intestines is prone to hematoma formation due to its proximity to the spinal column, particularly if a chance fracture occurs?
   a. ileum
   b. duodenum
   c. jejunum
   d. colon

6. Which organ, if injured, has the highest lethality in the field?
   a. liver
   b. pancreas
   c. kidneys
   d. aorta

7. Which of the following surrounds the abdominal organs?
   a. parietal viscera
   b. parietal peritoneum
   c. visceral viscera
   d. visceral peritoneum

8. Which of the following is NOT found in the abdominal cavity?
   a. pancreas
   b. cecum
   c. distal end of the esophagus
   d. spleen

9. Pain in the right shoulder may be referred pain from which of the following organs?
   a. spleen
   b. liver
   c. kidneys
   d. pancreas

10. The FAST exam does NOT ascertain the presence of blood in which of the following areas?
    a. right upper quadrant
    b. pelvis
    c. pericardium
    d. retroperitoneal

11. An injury to which organ may not present for 48 hours?
    a. spleen
    b. liver
    c. kidneys
    d. pancreas

12. Although all of the following organs are partially protected by the false ribs, which organ has the least protection?
    a. spleen
    b. liver
    c. kidneys
    d. pancreas

13. When the patient has pain at the costovertebral angle, injury to the _____ is suspected.
    a. spleen
    b. liver
    c. kidneys
    d. pancreas

14. Disruption of over 75% of the liver parenchyma is considered a grade _____ injury.
    a. I
    b. III
    c. V
    d. VII

15. Trauma causing the tunica albuginea to rupture will result in which of the following conditions?
    a. scrotal rupture
    b. penile fracture
    c. testicular dislocation
    d. coitus interruptus

Short Answer

Write a brief answer to each of the following questions.

16. How many liters of blood can be held in the abdominal cavity without visible abdominal distention?

_____

_____

17. What is FAST?

_____

_____

18. Describe the shearing injury of the liver.

_____

_____

19. What blunt trauma can cause injury to the pancreas?

_____

_____

20. Which solid organs can refer pain?

_____

_____

Fill in the Blank

Complete each sentence by adding the appropriate word in the provided blanks.

21. Diaphragmatic rupture most commonly occurs on the _____ side.

22. Blood in the urine is called _____ _____.

23. Hematomas between the surface of the organ and the visceral lining are called _____ _____.

24. _____ organ injury is responsible for hemorrhage and hypotension.

25. Back pain may be a sign of a _____ _____.

CHAPTER **7**

ORTHOPAEDIC TRAUMA

Case Study

Chief Concern

The call comes in as a collision at County Route 156 and Dexterville Road, an intersection that has become notorious for accidents. In fact, there was a fatal car crash just last week, and the county supervisor says the intersection is first on his list for realignment. The meeting point of County Route 156 and Dexterville Road is not really an intersection, but instead a bend in one road where it meets with the other. The only traffic control device is a yield sign. The highway design stems from the 1950s, and plans are underway to replace it with a modern roundabout.

Critical Thinking Questions

1. What are some of the possible orthopaedic trauma injuries that can be expected in the appendicular skeleton if the patient follows the up-and-over pathway?

   _____

   _____

2. What are some of the possible orthopaedic trauma injuries that can be expected in the appendicular skeleton if the patient follows the down-and-under pathway?

   _____

   _____

History

From down the road, Seth knows this is going to be a bad accident. Traffic is bottlenecked and the "light parade" is impressive. As he approaches the scene, he counts five patrol cars, a fire chief and deputy chief, an engine, and a heavy rescue, as well as fire police.

As predicted, one car T-boned the other, leaving the driver of the car struck in the driver's side pinned inside the car. Seth is directed to the patient being extricated. It seems her left hip is pinned under the door's armrest and her right hip is pinned under the armrest of the center console. Otherwise, she says she is fine. "Hard to believe she's fine," Seth thinks to himself as he looks at the 18-plus inches of intrusion into the driver's compartment.

Critical Thinking Questions

1. What are the important elements of the history that a Paramedic should obtain if the collision was truck versus car in the lateral impact?

   _____

   _____

2. What are the important elements of the history if the collision was car versus truck in the lateral impact?

_____

_____

Examination

The patient, Lydia, is speaking through a firefighter, via radio, who is inside the car with her as the extrication is in progress. Lydia says she had no loss of consciousness, no chest pain, no shortness of breath, and the only thing that hurts is her hips. Otherwise, Lydia says she is a healthy young woman with no past medical history, no medications, and no allergies.

As soon as the console is displaced, the Paramedics remove Lydia from the vehicle using a long axis drag. Almost immediately, she cries out in pain.

Critical Thinking Questions

1. What are the elements of the physical examination of a patient with suspected pelvic fracture?

_____

_____

2. Why is it inappropriate to "spring the hips"?

_____

_____

Assessment

An assessment of Lydia's injuries, performed in the relative privacy of the ambulance compartment, reveals Lydia is not incontinent of blood or urine, and she does not have ecchymosis along her flanks. However, she is complaining of lower back pain, along the lumbar–sacral line, but she denies any perineal numbness. "No saddle paresthesia," Seth thinks to himself as he proceeds to assess her femurs.

Critical Thinking Questions

1. What diagnosis did the Paramedic announce to the patient?

_____

_____

2. What are the possibilities of associated spinal injuries?

_____

_____

Treatment

Seth calls out to the EMT to obtain a pulse and blood pressure every five minutes while he and another EMT apply a pelvic sling. By sliding the sling under the patient's sacrum, Seth is able to secure the sling over her anterior superior iliac spine and ratchet it into place.

Critical Thinking Questions

1. What is the national standard of care of patients with suspected pelvic fractures?

_____

_____

2. Which of these devices would be useful if the patient developed hypotension secondary to internal hemorrhage from pelvic fractures?

_____

_____

Evaluation

"90 over 60 and her heart rate is 140 now," the EMT announces. Having already established one point of venous access, Seth prepares to start another one while advising the EMT to keep one eye on the patient's level of consciousness. "And let's step it up," he calls to the driver.

As he sits back in the bench seat, fastening the seat belt on, Seth thinks to himself, "Regional is only 10 minutes away. Hang in there, Lydia."

Critical Thinking Questions

1. What are some of the predictable complications associated with pelvic fractures?

_____

_____

2. What are some of the predictable complications associated with the treatments for sustained pelvic fractures?

_____

_____

Disposition

With lights flashing, the ambulance pulls into the ambulance bay at the regional trauma center. Fortunately, Seth used the camera on his phone to take a picture of the wreck. As they say, "A picture paints a thousand words." After one look at the crash scene, the chief of emergency services directs the patient into Trauma Bay One. Almost immediately, a swarm of people seem to appear from out of nowhere to assist.

Critical Thinking Questions

1. What is the most appropriate transport decision that will get the patient to definitive care?

_____

_____

2. What services does this patient need?

_____

_____

Practice Questions
Multiple Choice

Select the best answer for each of the following questions.

1. Which of the following forces "remodels" bone?
   a. tensile
   b. compressive
   c. torsion
   d. all of the above

2. Which of the following is NOT part of the female athlete's "triad"?
   a. depression
   b. anorexia
   c. amenorrhea
   d. osteoporosis

3. Loss of the integrity of a joint is called a _____ sprain.
   a. first degree
   b. partial
   c. complete
   d. fifth degree

4. What is the only point where the shoulder is directly attached to the axial skeleton?
   a. sternoclavicular joint
   b. acromioclavicular joint
   c. glenohumeral joint
   d. scapulothoracic joint

5. Which ligament connects the femur to the tibia and is needed so the knee does not "give out"?
   a. anterior cruciate
   b. posterior cruciate
   c. lateral collateral
   d. medial collateral

6. Which injury has been attributed to the "weekend warrior"?
   a. patellar tendon rupture
   b. Achilles tendon rupture
   c. quadriceps tendon rupture
   d. biceps tendon rupture

7. Which of the following dislocations results in the highest rate of neurovascular complications?
   a. elbow dislocation
   b. shoulder dislocation
   c. knee dislocation
   d. patellar dislocation

8. Which fracture is specific to children?
   a. Salter–Harris
   b. nursemaid's elbow
   c. Burkert
   d. Gustilo–Anderson

9. Which of the following is an ulna fracture with dislocation of the radioulnar joint?
   a. Galeazzi's fracture
   b. Monteggia's fracture
   c. Colles fracture
   d. chauffeur's fracture

10. When a patient falls on a flexed hand, with resultant displacement of the hand, it is a _____ fracture.
    a. Smith
    b. Colles
    c. hamate
    d. navicular

11. A jammed finger can result in a _____ fracture.
    a. Bennett's
    b. Mallet
    c. Smith
    d. Colles

12. Which of the following is NOT a mechanism for a pelvic fracture?
    a. lateral compression, T-bone MVC
    b. vertical shear, fall
    c. anterior compression, confined space cave-in
    d. posterior compression, rear-end MVC

13. Osteitis deformans, or Paget's disease, can cause pathological fractures of which bone?
    a. femur
    b. humerus
    c. pelvis
    d. hip

14. Which method of shoulder reduction is preferred for the elderly?
    a. Hippocratic
    b. Manes
    c. Stimson
    d. Kocher

15. What is a Velpeau bandage used to treat?
    a. shoulder dislocation
    b. elbow dislocation
    c. humerus fracture
    d. clavicular fracture

Short Answer

Write a brief answer to each of the following questions.

16. What complication is associated with the common scaphoid/navicular fracture?

_____

_____

17. Explain shin splints.

_____

_____

18. What is FACTS?

_____

_____

19. What is RICE?

_____

_____

20. What is compartment syndrome?

_____

_____

Fill in the Blank

Complete each sentence by adding the appropriate word in the provided blanks.

21. The study of forces exerted by muscles upon the skeleton is called _____.

22. If the tissue returns to its original shape following application of a force, it is called _____ deformity and no trauma is said to have occurred. If the tissue retains a new shape following application of a force, it is called _____ deformity and trauma has occurred.

23. Severe pain when a patient's arm is raised is suggestive of _____ _____ _____.

24. Although complete displacement of a bone out of joint is called a _____, a misalignment of the bone in a joint is called a _____.

25. For distal fractures of the forearm (radial and/or ulna), the _____ _____ _____ splint is useful.

CHAPTER 8

SOFT-TISSUE INJURY

Case Study

Chief Concern

"Meet the police, the corner of Dana and First Street, small child attacked by a pit bull terrier, multiple facial wounds," crackles the radio. Pulling a U-turn in the wide boulevard while the siren wails, the ambulance speeds off to the scene.

"Did you know there are over three-quarters of a million dog bites annually and the vast majority are by Rottweilers or pit bull terriers!?" Canon yells over the siren.

Critical Thinking Questions

1. What are some of the possible soft-tissue injuries that the Paramedic would suspect based on the mechanism of injury?

   _____

   _____

2. Are any of these soft-tissue injuries potentially life-threatening conditions?

   _____

   _____

History

The toddler is a "bloody mess," as blood seems to be seeping from multiple wounds. Apparently the child approached the dog through an open gate in a fence. When the dog started to growl, the child turned and ran away. The dog apparently closed the distance between them in an instant and attacked from behind. The dog continued to maul the toddler as he screamed. The driver of a passing car, seeing what was happening, stopped the car, and was able to drag the child away from the dog. The dog, at the end of his chain, continued to snap and bark.

Critical Thinking Questions

1. What are the important elements of the history that a Paramedic should obtain?

   _____

   _____

2. What are the confounding factors for wound healing?

   _____

   _____

Examination

Although the patient's facial wounds are impressive, Canon is more concerned with the gaping wound to the child's crown. Carefully probing the scalp with his gloved hands, he thinks he feels a step off. The child seems awake and alert, albeit a little upset, and appears to have no signs of a head injury.

"Let's get going," Canon announces. "Hold it, partner," an officer on scene retorts. "We need a statement and we need this little guy's home address so we can get ahold of his mother." Canon pulls the officer aside and explains that he thinks the child might have a life-threatening skull fracture. With that announcement, the officer clears a path through the crowd.

Critical Thinking Questions

1. What are the elements of the physical examination for soft-tissue injury?

   _____

   _____

2. What are the descriptions of the wounds?

   _____

   _____

Assessment

Despite the child's gruesome appearance, Canon tries to remain upbeat with the little boy. Although he appears calm, Canon knows that can change. He always keeps the ABCs foremost in his mind, despite the distraction of the wounds.

As the ambulance is about to depart, the rear doors fly open. The officer literally pushes the mother into the back of the ambulance and slams the doors while yelling, "Go, go, go!" The look on the mother's face says it all.

Critical Thinking Questions

1. What is the importance of making a determination of the type of wound?

   _____

   _____

2. What is the prognostic implication?

   _____

   _____

Treatment

"Yes," assures Canon. "I will answer all of your questions, but first I need to take care of your son." Canon busily applies sterile dressings to the obvious facial lacerations and then starts to wrap the patient's head with a bandage. Although he could have taken the time to decontaminate the child's wound, he knows that the hospital will do a better job.

Critical Thinking Questions

1. What is the national standard of care of patients with soft-tissue injuries?

   _____

   _____

2. Beyond initial first aid, what other care can be provided?

   _____

   _____

Evaluation

"Was the dog rabid?" asks the mother. Canon answers that they are not sure but that the animal control officer has taken control of the dog to test for rabies, if necessary.

Critical Thinking Questions

1. What are some of the predictable complications associated with dog bites?

   _____

   _____

2. What immunizations might the child receive?

   _____

   _____

Disposition

The mother insists on carrying her son into the emergency department where she is met by a nurse and directed into an open examination room. Canon insisted that the child be brought to the trauma center, not concerned about the facial wounds as much as he was concerned about the scalp laceration and an underlying linear skull fracture.

Critical Thinking Questions

1. What is the most appropriate transport decision that will get the patient to definitive care?

   _____

   _____

2. What are some of the transportation considerations?

   _____

   _____

Practice Questions
Multiple Choice

Select the best answer for each of the following questions.

1. What is the name for a wound that does not go below the dermis?
   a. abrasion
   b. laceration
   c. avulsion
   d. puncture

2. By definition, what area does a full thickness wound penetrate?
   a. deep fascia
   b. loose connective tissue
   c. dermis
   d. superficial fascia

3. What is the most commonly amputated appendage?
    a. fingers
    b. hand
    c. toes
    d. feet

4. Which of the following wounds tends to bleed the least?
    a. partial amputation
    b. laceration
    c. partial avulsion
    d. complete amputation

5. When does a wound start to contract?
    a. hemostasis stage
    b. proliferative phase
    c. granulation
    d. neovascularization

6. A partial thickness wound that affects the epidermis but does not extend into the dermis layer is a stage _____ pressure sore.
    a. one
    b. two
    c. three
    d. four

7. Which method of wound closure is useful in battlefield/wilderness situations for deep wounds?
    a. sutures
    b. staples
    c. skin glue
    d. Steri-strips

8. Which medications have been implicated in delayed wound healing?
    a. corticosteroids
    b. anticoagulants
    c. NSAIDs
    d. all of the above

9. Which medical conditions have been implicated in delayed wound healing?
    a. COPD
    b. HIV
    c. diabetes
    d. all of the above

10. What is a sunken eyeball that may represent an orbital fracture called?
    a. epiphthalmos
    b. enophthalmos
    c. esophthalmos
    d. exophthalmos

11. Bloody wound drainage is documented as _____.
    a. serous
    b. sanguineous
    c. serosanguineous
    d. purulent

12. What is wound drainage that does not soak through a single-layer thickness dressing called?
    a. scant
    b. small
    c. minor
    d. trivial

13. What animal is responsible for the majority of animal bites?
    a. raccoons
    b. ferrets
    c. cats
    d. dogs

14. Which of the following is a hemostatic agent made from minerals?
    a. zeolite
    b. chitin
    c. chitosan
    d. fibrin

15. What is the procedure of choice for severe uncontrolled arterial bleeding?
    a. standard pressure dressing
    b. Israeli trauma bandage
    c. tourniquet
    d. pressure points

Short Answer

Write a brief answer to each of the following questions.

16. What is primary and secondary wound healing?

_____

_____

17. What causes death from crush injury on scene, and what causes death days later?

_____

_____

18. What is the MESS?

_____

_____

19. How do topical antibiotics work?

_____

_____

20. What is a bioengineered skin equivalent?

_____

_____

Fill in the Blank

Complete each sentence by adding the appropriate word in the provided blanks.

21. A raised prominent scar, called a _____ scar, can result in _____.

22. Langer's lines are called _____ _____ lines, whereas Kraissl's lines are _____ _____ lines.

23. A nonsterile _____ holds the sterile _____ in place.

24. Risk for decubitus ulcer formation is determined in the long-term care industry using the _____ _____ _____ _____.

25. Limbs pinned under debris from a collapsed building are at risk for _____ injury, a form of _____ injury.

CHAPTER 9

BURN TRAUMA

Case Study

Chief Concern

"Burns from anhydrous ammonia," is the report. The first responders from the local volunteer fire department, many of them local farmers, are already on scene. The chatter on the police band radio states the "perps" were caught "pink-handed." Local farmers have been using a new product that stains the anhydrous ammonia pink. It serves a twofold purpose. Not only does it help them identify leaks, but it also leaves stains on the hands of thieves.

Apparently, the thief had tried to tap a nurse tank. Fortunately for him, a passing motorist on the way to church detected the odor, saw the suspicious vehicle, and called police who, in turn, called EMS for the patient.

The farmer, whose house was over a quarter of a mile away, had to be taken to the hospital by ambulance for "complications" that arose from exposure to the ammonia.

Critical Thinking Questions

1. What is anhydrous ammonia?

   _____
   _____

2. Why is anhydrous ammonia stolen?

   _____
   _____

History

The patient is "in extremis" when the Paramedics arrive. Apparently, he had taken a whiff of the anhydrous ammonia and now he is having a "coughing fit." Between his coughing fits, the patient has a loud audible wheeze.

Firefighters have already tried to put oxygen on him, but he swats them away, preferring to run, stop, go to all fours, cough, and get up to repeat it again. The firefighters elect to "irrigate" the patient with a fog stream from the fire hose. The patient has already stripped prior to their arrival.

Critical Thinking Questions

1. What are the important elements of the history that a Paramedic should obtain?

   _____
   _____

2. What is the symptom pattern associated with exposure to anhydrous ammonia?

   _____
   _____

Examination

Starting with the upper airway, the Paramedic works methodically down the chest. Stridor is appreciated in the upper airway, and the Paramedic hears a loud bronchial wheeze as well. The base of the lungs remains clear. "Good," the Paramedic thinks. "As long as we can keep the airway open, he can get oxygen."

Critical Thinking Questions

1. What are the elements of the physical examination of a patient with suspected toxic exposure?

_____

_____

2. Why is a respiratory examination a critical element in this examination?

_____

_____

Assessment

Finally, the firefighters are able to wrestle the patient to the ground and get him some oxygen. The oxygen seems to give the patient some relief and he becomes less combative.

Above the din of the firefighters, the Paramedic explains to the patient what he is going to do for him. The patient, a twentysomething man, seems relieved that relief is on the way.

Critical Thinking Questions

1. What is the assessment of the patient's condition?

_____

_____

2. What are the initial priorities of care based on the Paramedic's assessment?

_____

_____

Treatment

Utilizing the conscious sedation algorithm, the Paramedics elect to sedate. They intubate the patient using an extra large endotracheal tube. This permits more careful monitoring of his oxygenation and ensures he has a patent airway.

Critical Thinking Questions

1. What is the initial care of patients with exposure to anhydrous ammonia?

_____

_____

2. What is the focus of care of patients with exposure to anhydrous ammonia?

_____

_____

Evaluation

Since the patient is finally intubated, the Paramedic can assess the patient for other injuries. The first signs of injury are the patient's fluorescent pink hands. Apparently, the anhydrous ammonia must have somehow gotten on his hands. Looking carefully, the Paramedic can see the remains of his leather gloves, which must have been frozen to the patient's hands and literally peeled off when the burning got intense.

Critical Thinking Questions

1. What are the visible effects seen with a topical exposure to anhydrous ammonia?

_____

_____

2. What are the effects of topical exposure to anhydrous ammonia that are not visible?

_____

_____

Disposition

The firefighters had called for air medical support almost immediately upon their arrival, and almost immediately they were denied. The dispatcher explains that any patient exposed to hazardous materials can be a danger to the flight crew; in this case, ammonia off-gassing in the confined space of the helicopter can be devastating to the air crew.

Critical Thinking Questions

1. What is the most appropriate transport decision that will get the patient to definitive care?

_____

_____

2. Why is the appropriate transportation decision important?

_____

_____

Practice Questions
Multiple Choice

Select the best answer for each of the following questions.

1. What is the most common chemical exposure?
   a. lime
   b. drain cleaner
   c. bleach
   d. sodium hydroxide

2. Which of the following processes does NOT result in liquefaction necrosis?
   a. dissolving
   b. saponification
   c. dessication
   d. denaturing

3. Which of the following is an alkali?
   a. phenol
   b. hydrofluoric acid
   c. anhydrous ammonia
   d. white phosphorus

4. What term is used to describe the amount of electricity?
   a. amperage
   b. voltage
   c. ohms
   d. current

5. What term is used to describe the speed of alternating current?
   a. milliamperes
   b. hertz
   c. volts
   d. ohms

6. What is the best source of information for emergency care on the scene of a chemical spill?
   a. material safety data sheet
   b. emergency response guidebook
   c. compendium of chemicals
   d. national formulary

7. What type of burn extends just slightly into the dermis?
   a. superficial burn
   b. partial thickness burn
   c. full thickness burn
   d. terminal burn

8. The outermost ring of burn is generally superficial and is called the zone of _____.
   a. hyperemia
   b. stasis
   c. coagulation
   d. necrosis

9. What is the preferred method of burn estimation?
   a. rule of nines
   b. modified rule of nines
   c. Lund–Browder chart
   d. palmar rule

10. Which of the following is NOT an early sign of carbon monoxide poisoning?
    a. headache
    b. confusion
    c. nausea and vomiting
    d. combativeness

11. Overly aggressive fluid resuscitation of burns can lead to fluid creep and all of the following complications EXCEPT _____.
    a. increased burn edema formation
    b. abdominal compartment syndrome
    c. increased intracranial pressure
    d. acute respiratory distress

12. What is the most effective means of pain management?
    a. sterile dressings
    b. morphine IM
    c. fentanyl IN
    d. diazepam IV

13. A Paramedic will use calcium gluconate to treat burns from which of the following substances?
    a. hydrofluoric acid
    b. anhydrous ammonia
    c. calcium oxide
    d. phenol

14. A Paramedic will use vegetable oil to treat burns from which of the following substances?
    a. hydrofluoric acid
    b. anhydrous ammonia
    c. calcium oxide
    d. phenol

15. Which of the following is NOT a criteria for burn center admission?
    a. full thickness burn over 5%
    b. inhalation burns
    c. burns and trauma
    d. hands or feet burned

Short Answer

Write a brief answer to each of the following questions.

16. Describe an emergency escharotomy.

    _____

    _____

17. Describe signs of smoke inhalation.

    _____

    _____

18. Describe the actions of hydroxocobalamin.

    _____

    _____

19. Describe fluid creep.

    _____

    _____

20. What is the Parkland formula?

    _____

    _____

Fill in the Blank

Complete each sentence by adding the appropriate word in the provided blanks.

21. The process of denaturing proteins in heat is called _____.

22. Whereas acids cause _____ necrosis, alkalis cause _____ necrosis.

23. Skin is a _____ and does not naturally allow the passage of electricity easily.

24. A stress ulcer that develops after an electric shock is called a _____ _____.

25. The _____ _____ is used for ocular burns.

CHAPTER 10

PEDIATRIC TRAUMA CONSIDERATIONS

Case Study

Chief Concern

"Ouch!" is all anyone heard when the nine-year-old boy, Dwayne, hit the ground. The four-foot boy had climbed up the apple tree at least 12 feet when the branch snapped and he came tumbling down.

A concerned neighbor, watching the boys climbing in the old apple tree, immediately called emergency services before running out. The boys are clustered around Dwayne, who is holding his head and moaning.

Critical Thinking Questions

1. What are some of the potentially life-threatening injuries that Dwayne sustained?

   _____

   _____

2. What other secondary injuries could the child have sustained?

   _____

   _____

History

As the fire department Paramedics arrive, the mother runs to her son's side. "What happened?" she implores the Paramedics. The pumper's lieutenant gently redirects the mother to the side to permit the Paramedics room to work on her son.

"Mom," the Paramedic asks, "could you please tell me about your son?" She explains that her son is a healthy young boy without any allergies or medical problems. In fact, the only medicine he takes is some vitamins.

As the mother explains the boy's medical history, the vigilant Paramedic overhears the conversation and makes mental notes as she proceeds with the physical examination. "Where does it hurt?" she asks. The boy grabs his head and moans.

Critical Thinking Questions

1. What are the important elements of the history that a Paramedic should obtain?

   _____

   _____

2. What additional information would be helpful?

   _____

   _____

Examination

With manual stabilization of the patient's head in place, the Paramedic proceeds to perform both a primary and secondary assessment. Of primary concern is the rapidly developing "egg" on the patient's forehead, his complaint of head pain, and the speed of his response to questions. Although there is no drainage from the ears or nose, or any postauricular ecchymosis, the Paramedic starts to focus the examination on the potential for traumatic brain injury.

Critical Thinking Questions

1. What are the elements of the physical examination of a pediatric trauma patient?

_____

_____

2. Why is a cranial nerve exam a critical element in this examination?

_____

_____

Assessment

"What's going on? What's happening to my son?!" implores the mother. The Paramedic quietly explains that her son may have hit his head on the ground and that he needs to go to the hospital immediately. The mother's only question is, "Can I ride with him?"

Critical Thinking Questions

1. What diagnosis did the Paramedic announce to the patient's mother?

_____

_____

2. Based on the patient's age, is it appropriate to discuss the diagnosis with the patient?

_____

_____

Treatment

After securely immobilizing the child to a pediatric backboard, which is in turn secured to a full-length backboard, the "package" is loaded onto the stretcher. With continuous high-flow, high-concentration oxygen in place, the Paramedic keeps a vigilant eye on the boy's mental status. If any further decline is noted, she is prepared to intubate him if needed.

Critical Thinking Questions

1. What is the national standard of care of patients with suspected traumatic brain injury?

_____

_____

2. How should this patient be positioned on the stretcher?

_____

_____

Evaluation

While aboard the ambulance, the boy's breathing seems to become much more labored and his blood pressure drops. Although the Paramedic anticipates a change in the respiratory pattern, the blood pressure should be going up, not down. A falling blood pressure generally means that the patient is bleeding somewhere internally.

Starting at the head and moving down, the Paramedic carefully assesses the boy. "Diminished breath sounds!" she exclaims. Of course, she thinks to herself, he must have hit his ribs on a branch on the way down to the ground.

Critical Thinking Questions

1. What are some of the predictable complications associated with pediatric chest trauma?

_____

_____

2. What are some other predictable complications based on the mechanism of injury?

_____

_____

Disposition

After decompressing the patient's collapsed lung, the blood pressure returns and the boy's breathing becomes easier. Making a mental note of the procedure, the Paramedic continues her assessment as they arrive at the trauma center until she is satisfied that all injuries can be accounted for.

Critical Thinking Questions

1. Does Dwayne's mechanism of injury meet major trauma criteria?

_____

_____

2. What is the most appropriate transport decision that will get the patient to definitive care?

_____

_____

Practice Questions

Multiple Choice

Select the best answer for each of the following questions.

1. Which of the following is NOT a common source of injury among children 0 to 1 year of age?
   a. child abuse
   b. burns
   c. motor vehicle crashes
   d. drowning

2. Extremity injuries are NOT common in which of the following situations?
   a. pedestrian versus motor vehicle
   b. falls
   c. bicycle crashes
   d. gunshot wounds

3. Which of the following is NOT included in Waddell's triad of pediatric injury following impact with a motor vehicle?
   a. femur fractures
   b. chest injury
   c. head injury
   d. back injury

4. Generally, a serious pediatric fall is defined as a fall from what distance?
   a. two or more stories
   b. three times the child's height
   c. six feet
   d. standing position

5. Head injury in a shaken baby scenario is likely to be caused by which of the following conditions?
   a. epidural hematoma
   b. subdural hematoma
   c. subarachnoid hemorrhage
   d. diffuse axonal injury

6. Commotio cordis is a chest injury that results in what condition?
   a. fractured ribs
   b. flail segment
   c. pneumothorax
   d. ventricular fibrillation

7. Which fractures are seen almost exclusively in children?
   a. greenstick
   b. spiral
   c. compound
   d. transverse

8. Which fractures involve the growth plate?
   a. Salter–Harris
   b. buckle
   c. greenstick
   d. spiral

9. Which of the following does NOT meet the physiologic criteria for transportation to the pediatric trauma center?
   a. Glasgow Coma Scale less than 14
   b. systolic blood pressure less than (70 + 2 × age)
   c. respiratory rate 10 and > 29 if older than 1 year
   d. heart rate greater than 120 beats per minute

10. Which of the following injuries does NOT meet the anatomic injury criteria for transportation to the pediatric trauma center?
    a. fractured ribs
    b. flail chest
    c. fractured pelvis
    d. mangled extremity

11. Which of the following does NOT meet the mechanism of injury criteria for transportation to the pediatric trauma center?
    a. fall of three times the child's height
    b. motorcycle crash at speeds greater than 20 miles per hour
    c. ejection from the motor vehicle
    d. car versus pedestrian at five miles per hour

12. What is the typical fluid bolus for a child in shock?
    a. 10 mL/kg
    b. 20 mL/kg
    c. 250 mL
    d. 1,000 mL

13. What is an excellent indicator of shock in children?
    a. blood pressure
    b. heart rate
    c. capillary refill
    d. respiratory rate

14. What is the best estimate of burn surface area in children?
    a. rule of nines
    b. modified rule of nines
    c. Lund–Browder chart
    d. palmar method

15. What is the most commonly injured abdominal organ in children?
    a. spleen
    b. kidneys
    c. liver
    d. pancreas

Short Answer

Write a brief answer to each of the following questions.

16. Describe SCIWORA.

_____

_____

17. What is a stinger?

_____

_____

18. How does a blow to the chest cause sudden cardiac death?

_____

_____

19. Describe how a greenstick fracture occurs.

_____

_____

20. Describe how a buckle fracture occurs.

_____

_____

Fill in the Blank

Complete each sentence by adding the appropriate word in the provided blanks.

21. Seizures following trauma are called _____ _____ _____.

22. Pediatric spinal injury that does not show up on X-ray is called _____.

23. Sudden cardiac death following a blow to the chest is called _____ _____.

24. A fracture that occurs when the bone bends, but does not break, is called a _____ fracture.

25. Fractures involving the growth plate are called _____ _____ fractures.

CHAPTER 11

TRAUMA RESUSCITATION

Case Study

The police have already cut the patient down by the time the Paramedics arrive. The patient reportedly has a thready carotid pulse and resembles a rag doll lying on the floor, with limbs strewn about in no particular manner or reason.

"Twentysomething," guesses the first Paramedic as she places the patient's head in a neutral in-line position. The ligature marks on the throat are distinctive, red angry bands across the trachea just above the Adam's apple.

Critical Thinking Questions

1. What are some of the possible life-threatening injuries that would be suspected based on the mechanism of injury?

_____

_____

2. What else should the Paramedic suspect?

_____

_____

Fortunately, the airway is patent to the cords and the Paramedic is able to pass the endotracheal tube easily and without resistance. The patient is manually ventilated with the tube in place until his end-tidal carbon dioxide levels return to normal. As a result of that action, the patient's pulses become stronger. However, the patient remains unconscious.

Critical Thinking Questions

3. What is the most appropriate transport decision that will get the patient to definitive care?

_____

_____

4. What are some of the transportation considerations?

_____

_____

Practice Questions

Multiple Choice

Select the best answer for each of the following questions.

1. Which of the following is NOT a form of distributive shock?
   a. spinal shock
   b. hemorrhagic shock
   c. septic shock
   d. anaphylactic shock

2. What is the first response to hypovolemia?
   a. baroreceptor-mediated vasoconstriction
   b. adrenal-mediated vasoconstriction
   c. chemoreceptor-mediated vasoconstriction
   d. antidiuretic hormone-mediated vasoconstriction

3. The most sensitive chemoreceptors to carbon dioxide (acidosis) are in which part of the body?
   a. medulla oblongata
   b. carotid
   c. aorta
   d. cerebral cortex

4. Decompensation can occur because of which of the following conditions?
   a. loss of epinephrine-mediated vasoconstriction
   b. acidosis that causes vasodilation
   c. relaxation of the systemic circulation
   d. all of the above

5. What may cause altered mental status?
   a. hypoxia
   b. hypotension
   c. head injury
   d. all of the above

6. In which of the following situations should a surgical airway NOT be used?
   a. massive mandible trauma
   b. unrecognizable facial anatomy
   c. crushed trachea
   d. aspiration

7. In the face of a simple pneumothorax, what is likely to be the most dependable sign of a developing tension pneumothorax?
   a. decreased pulse oximeter
   b. hypotension
   c. jugular venous distention
   d. hyperresonant percussion

8. Where is a needle thoracostomy for a tension pneumothorax on the right side performed?
   a. fifth ICS at the left MCL
   b. second ICS at the left MCL
   c. fifth ICS at the right MCL
   d. second ICS at the right MCL

9. What is the clinical presentation for the patient with neurogenic shock?
   a. warm and pink below the level of injury
   b. cool and pale below the level of the injury
   c. warm and pink above the level of the injury
   d. none of the above

10. What is the most effective means of controlling arterial bleeding?
    a. direct pressure
    b. tourniquet
    c. elevation
    d. pressure point

11. Which of the following is an argument for permissive hypotension?
    a. Lower blood pressures permit clot formation.
    b. Hemodilution by overly aggressive fluids leads to coagulopathy.
    c. Overly aggressive fluid resuscitation leads to acute respiratory distress syndrome.
    d. All of the above.

12. Which of the following is NOT a clinical endpoint for fluid resuscitation?
    a. palpable radial pulse
    b. mean arterial pressure of 60 mmHg
    c. systolic blood pressure of 120 mmHg
    d. appropriate mentation

13. As little as _____ mL of fluid is thought to dilute clotting factors.
    a. 250
    b. 500
    c. 750
    d. 1,000

14. What is the treatment of choice for neurogenic shock?
    a. fluid resuscitation
    b. dobutamine
    c. norepinephrine
    d. dopamine

15. What is the treatment for patients with adrenal insufficiency who are in shock?
    a. methylprednisolone
    b. dobutamine
    c. fluid resuscitation
    d. furosemide

Short Answer

Write a brief answer to each of the following questions.

16. Explain nitrogen washout.

_____

_____

17. Explain permissive hypotension.

_____

_____

18. Explain how to use a blood pressure cuff as a tourniquet.

_____

_____

19. Explain the pathophysiology of neurogenic shock.

_____

_____

20. What is the contraindication to nasal intubation of a trauma patient?

_____

_____

Fill in the Blank

Complete each sentence by adding the appropriate word in the provided blanks.

21. Blood pressure is sensed by _____.

22. Another name for the flutter valve used for a pneumothorax is a _____ _____.

23. Purposely maintaining a patient's blood pressure low is called _____ _____.

24. A maximum of _____ intubation attempts is recommended before a _____ _____ is used.

25. The _____ system is responsible for the production of red blood cells.

CHAPTER 12

HEAT EMERGENCIES

Case Study

Chief Concern

The headline of the local paper states, "Hottest summer on record." Glenn huffs as he wipes the sweat off his brow and says, "Like that's news." His homily on heat is interrupted by the siren. As he scrambles to the rig, the speaker announces that a 29-year-old migrant worker has collapsed at the local orchard. The orchard is known for hiring migrant labor to help with the harvest.

The dispatcher continues the report, stating that the patient is conscious but confused and that local police units are also en route to assist.

Critical Thinking Questions

1. What are some of the possible causes of the patient's syncope?

_____

_____

2. Of these possibilities, which is potentially a life-threatening condition?

_____

_____

History

It is a sweltering hot late summer day. Although the temperature is only 96°F, the humidity is 60% and climbing. This group of fruit pickers had just started the season but had been working hard all week, basically from sunup to sundown. Emanuel had just arrived to camp. His wife was sick and he had to stay back for a few days to help with the children, so he is trying to make up for lost time.

Critical Thinking Questions

1. What are the important elements of the history that a Paramedic should obtain?

_____

_____

2. What medications interfere with a person's ability to dissipate heat?

_____

_____

Examination

Emanuel is confused, his speech is slurred, and his vital signs are "hyperdynamic." With his heart racing to keep up, Glenn knows that he is vasodilating. "I could put a 16 into his jugular from across the room," he declares.

Critical Thinking Questions

1. What are the elements of the physical examination of a patient with suspected heatstroke?

_____

_____

2. Why is a 12-lead ECG a critical element in this examination?

_____

_____

Assessment

The patient is "hot as a pistol," Glenn notes. However, he is still sweating. Glenn knows better than to fall into that trap. "He's having a heatstroke," Glenn states. "Let's get him out of the sun, into the ambulance, and let's get his clothes off of him. Say, does anyone have any ice?"

Critical Thinking Questions

1. What diagnosis did the Paramedic announce?

_____

_____

2. What was the key element of this diagnosis?

_____

_____

Treatment

With the air conditioning blasting, the crew starts to place ice packs in the patient's armpits and groin. Suddenly, Glenn sticks his head out of the patient compartment and yells out to the crowd of workers, "Hey, anybody got one of those bottle sprayers that's empty?"

Critical Thinking Questions

1. What is the national standard of care of patients with suspected heat illness?

_____

_____

2. What is the therapeutic goal of cooling the patient?

_____

_____

Evaluation

Suddenly, Emanuel starts to seize. Glenn knows that seizures are a predictable complication and is prepared. Almost as soon as the tonic phase is over, Glenn prepares the intranasal midazolam. For two or three minutes, which seem like an eternity to Glenn, Emanuel continues to seize and his temperature continues to climb.

Critical Thinking Questions

1. What are some of the predictable complications associated with hyperthermia?

_____

_____

2. What are some of the predictable complications associated with the treatment of hyperthermia?

_____

_____

Disposition

As the seizure abates, the ambulance pulls into the hospital. Unloading the patient, Glenn smiles. He has managed to intubate the patient, start two IVs, cool the patient with ice packs and a mist bottle, monitor the patient's ECG, and obtain a 12-lead ECG.

Critical Thinking Questions

1. What is the most appropriate transport decision that will get the patient to definitive care?

_____

_____

2. What are some of the transportation considerations?

_____

_____

Practice Questions

Multiple Choice

Select the best answer for each of the following questions.

1. What organ plays a key role in thermoregulation?
   a. hypothalamus
   b. medulla oblongata
   c. spleen
   d. kidneys

2. Which receptors stimulate the production of sweat?
   a. alpha
   b. beta
   c. cholinergic
   d. muscarinic

3. What delineates heat exhaustion from heatstroke in the field?
   a. syncope
   b. anhydrosis
   c. temperature
   d. diaphoresis

4. What symptom differentiates salt depletion heat exhaustion from water depletion heat exhaustion?
   a. vomiting
   b. temperature
   c. level of consciousness
   d. orthostatic hypotension

5. What key symptom can differentiate heat exhaustion from heat fatigue in the field?
   a. orthostatic hypotension
   b. tachycardia
   c. muscle cramps
   d. difficulty with fine motor skills

6. What differentiates exertional heatstroke from nonexertional heatstroke?
   a. anhydrosis
   b. level of consciousness
   c. temperature
   d. orthostatic hypotension

7. Which of the following is NOT part of the classic heatstroke triad?
   a. altered mental status
   b. anhydrosis
   c. vomiting
   d. hyperthermia

8. Which of the following is NOT an indicator of malignant hyperthermia?
   a. masseter muscle spasm
   b. hypercarbia
   c. muscle rigidity
   d. hypoxia

9. What is an increase in body temperature induced by a fever called?
   a. hyperthermia
   b. hyperpyrexia
   c. hyperpituitaria
   d. hypersympathetic stimulation

10. Which of the following is NOT a potential indicator of heatstroke in an infected patient?
    a. syncope
    b. anticholinergics
    c. seizure
    d. hypotension

11. Which of the following hormonal disorders does NOT cause heatstroke?
    a. thyrotoxic crisis
    b. pheochromocytoma
    c. diabetes
    d. Graves' disease

12. What is the key symptom that is most common in the vast majority of heatstroke illnesses, regardless of etiology?
    a. sudden onset of altered mental status
    b. sudden increase in respiratory rate
    c. sudden drop in blood pressure
    d. sudden increase in temperature

13. What is the key hemodynamic factor that indicates heatstroke?
    a. dropping mean arterial pressure
    b. sustained tachycardia
    c. development of jugular venous distention
    d. widening pulse pressure

14. What is an electrocardiographic indicator of heatstroke?
    a. global ST elevation
    b. inverted T waves
    c. development of Q waves
    d. reverse R to R progression

15. What is the most effective means of cooling a patient?
    a. evaporative techniques
    b. strategic ice packing
    c. ice water immersion
    d. iced gastric lavage/gavage

Short Answer

Write a brief answer to each of the following questions.

16. Describe the mechanism that causes heat syncope.

   _____

   _____

17. What is the "triple impact" of hyperthermia on oxygenation?

   _____

   _____

18. Describe an evaporative technique for cooling the body.

   _____

   _____

19. What is heat-related rhabdomyolysis?

   _____

   _____

20. What are the early signs of hyponatremia?

   _____

   _____

Fill in the Blank

Complete each sentence by adding the appropriate word in the provided blanks.

21. Loss of heat by evaporation is called _____.

22. The table that combines heat with humidity to create a "perceived" heat is called the _____ _____.

23. Excessive water intake to ward off heat exhaustion can lead to _____ _____.

24. Temporary loss of consciousness due to heat-induced vasodilation is called _____ _____.

25. Absence of sweat in the face of heat is called _____.

CHAPTER 13

COLD EMERGENCIES

Case Study

Chief Concern

The day is crisp, cold, and beautiful, a perfect day to go cross-country skiing. However, the two skiers realize they have pushed themselves too hard. The short winter day is starting to wane and they are still miles from their vehicle. Pushing on, they arrive at the car after dark. Wet, cold, and hungry, the skiers jump into the car only to find it has a dead battery.

Local police, as part of their routine patrol, check all of the trailheads after dark to see if any vehicles have been left behind. As an officer goes down the unimproved road, one of the skiers appears in his headlights. "Thank God you are here!" he exclaims. "Our battery is dead. Can you help?"

After stowing the man's skis in the trunk, the pair drives to the trailhead at the end of the road. The police officer finds the passenger, Saniyah, huddled under an old oil tarp, shivering and afraid. After a few questions, she seems confused. EMS is dispatched.

Critical Thinking Questions

1. What problems might the skier be experiencing?

   _____

   _____

2. What factors may have led to this problem?

   _____

   _____

History

Saniyah is shivering and complains of feeling "cold in her bones." The officer is having a hard time understanding her, as her words are slurred. He asks if she has been drinking. She adamantly denies she has been drinking until her boyfriend reminds her of the wine they shared on the trail.

"Let's get you into the warm patrol car," suggests the officer. As Saniyah is assisted to the car, she stumbles several times. The officer notes that her clothing is stiff and frozen. "Do you have a change of clothes?" he asks.

Critical Thinking Questions

1. What are the important elements of the history that a Paramedic should obtain?

   _____

   _____

2. What role does age play in the problem of cold illness?

_____

_____

Examination

After finding Saniyah in the back seat of the patrol car huddled with her boyfriend, the Paramedic proceeds to perform his physical exam, focusing on her temperature. The tympanic membrane thermometer reads 90°F (32°C).

Fortunately, Saniyah is still shivering. "Let's get in the back of the ambulance and out of those cold, wet clothes," the Paramedic suggests. "Someone get the extra blankets from under the bench seat."

Critical Thinking Questions

1. What are the elements of the physical examination of a patient with suspected cold-related illness?

_____

_____

2. Why should a careful neurological examination be performed?

_____

_____

Assessment

Saniyah's vital signs indicate she is hyperdynamic. "That's to be expected," the Paramedic announces. "Let's get moving, slowly, toward the hospital." Saniyah's pupils are so dilated that the Paramedic cannot tell if they are reactive.

"How is she?" her boyfriend asks from the front seat. "She will be fine," replies the Paramedic. "It's just a case of exposure."

Critical Thinking Questions

1. What level of hypothermia is this patient experiencing?

_____

_____

2. What key finding suggests that the patient has progressed in her illness?

_____

_____

Treatment

The Paramedic methodically undresses the patient, assessing the needed portion of her body, then covering her to protect her modesty. He cuts up her sleeves to expose her arms for vital signs, then wraps the arm with a dry towel. Next, he cuts open her shirt, places the electrodes, then covers her with a blanket. He deliberately works head-to-toe, assessing her neurological function and checking pulses as he goes.

Critical Thinking Questions

1. What is the national standard of care of patients with suspected mild hypothermia?

_____

_____

2. What are some of the patient-specific concerns and considerations that the Paramedic should consider when applying this plan of care that is intended to treat a broad patient population presenting with mild hypothermia?

_____

_____

Evaluation

Stripped of her wet clothes and resting under a pile of warm blankets, Saniyah appears to be falling asleep. The Paramedic seems satisfied that things are going well until he realizes that she may not be asleep. "Saniyah, Saniyah," the Paramedic calls as he gently shakes her. She is arousable but is very slow to respond. More importantly, the Paramedic realizes that Saniyah has stopped shivering under the blankets.

Critical Thinking Questions

1. What could have led to this event?

_____

_____

2. What would be the treatment for this change to moderate hypothermia?

_____

_____

Disposition

Saniyah is transported to the local critical access point where the physician assistant has already created a satellite link with the trauma center. "Be careful," the attending from the regional hospital warns. "Rough handling can put her into cardiac arrest. However, it sounds like from the medic's report that you should be able to care for her. I will keep this link open in case she is worse than reported and may need intensive care."

Critical Thinking Questions

1. What is the most appropriate transport decision that will get the patient to definitive care?

_____

_____

2. What are some of the transportation considerations?

_____

_____

Practice Questions
Multiple Choice

Select the best answer for each of the following questions.

1. Through what process is the majority of body heat lost?
   a. radiation
   b. evaporation
   c. conduction
   d. convection

2. In which situation is heat lost most quickly?
   a. standing in front of a fan
   b. sitting covered in snow
   c. standing while doused with water
   d. sitting immersed in water

3. What part of the body controls the core temperature?
   a. medulla oblongata
   b. brainstem
   c. cerebellum
   d. hypothalamus

4. What state are muscles in when they use up all of their energy stores?
   a. glycogen debt
   b. extreme fatigue
   c. myocellular failure
   d. anaerobic metabolism

5. Pulmonary hypertension, and subsequent right-sided heart failure, is primarily due to what cause?
   a. pulmonary vasoconstriction
   b. oxyhemoglobin dissociation
   c. cardiovascular collapse
   d. cold diuresis

6. Which of the following is a local cold injury?
   a. frostbite
   b. trench foot
   c. frostnip
   d. all of the above

7. Which of the following is NOT a sign of altered mental status secondary to malfunction of the hypothalamus?
   a. shivering
   b. paradoxical undressing
   c. terminal burrowing
   d. irritability

8. Which of the following is NOT part of the negative impact of alcohol on hypothermia?
   a. misguided sense of well-being
   b. increased vasodilation
   c. depression of shivering
   d. impaired judgment

9. What ECG sign is pathognomonic for hypothermia?
   a. serial T wave inversion
   b. global ST segment depression
   c. appearance of J wave
   d. widened QT interval

10. Which of the following pupillary changes will NOT be seen with hypothermia?
    a. sluggish
    b. dilated
    c. constricted
    d. fixed

11. Which of the following patient actions will indicate to the Paramedic to begin active external rewarming?
    a. shows impaired judgment
    b. is hyperdynamic
    c. stops shivering
    d. has fine motor impairment

12. Which of the following patient actions will indicate to the Paramedic to begin active internal rewarming?
    a. becomes unconscious
    b. is hypodynamic
    c. has altered mental status
    d. stops shivering

13. Encouraging thermogenesis with warm blankets is an example of which type of rewarming?
    a. active external rewarming
    b. passive external rewarming
    c. active internal rewarming
    d. passive internal rewarming

14. Which of the following is NOT an acceptable source of external heat?
    a. heat lamps directed toward the body
    b. chemical heat packs placed directly on the skin
    c. hot water bottles in the groin and axilla
    d. prewarmed blankets draped over the body

15. What is usually the first dysrhythmia to present in the patient with hypothermia?
    a. atrial fibrillation
    b. bradycardia
    c. pulseless electrical activity
    d. ventricular fibrillation

Short Answer

Write a brief answer to each of the following questions.

16. What is cold diuresis?

_____

_____

17. Describe the mechanism that creates trench foot.

_____

_____

18. List the "umbles."

_____

_____

19. Describe the "after drop" phenomenon.

_____

_____

20. Describe rewarming shock.

_____

_____

Fill in the Blank

Complete each sentence by adding the appropriate word in the provided blanks.

21. The _____ _____ _____ takes both temperature and wind speed into account when calculating the perceived temperature.

22. Shivering is an example of _____.

23. A large volume of dilute urine is the result of _____ _____.

24. The Osborne wave is another name for a _____ wave.

25. Loss of core temperature with external rewarming is called _____ _____ _____.

CHAPTER **14**

MOUNTAIN MEDICINE

Case Study

Chief Concern

Jay is particularly thrilled about registering for the Pikes Peak Marathon. An almost 6,000 feet gain in altitude, with the last 2,000 feet in the last three miles, the race is a true test of endurance; heck, sometimes it even snows during the run. At over 12,000 feet, Pikes Peak is the ultimate challenge to the conditioned athlete, so Jay left from MacArthur Airport at Islip, Long Island, his hometown, and flew to Colorado.

Jay figures if he can run up Mt. Elbert (elevation 14,433 feet), the highest mountain in the lower 48 states (except Mt. Whitney in California), he can easily challenge the shorter Pikes Peak. Excited to be in Colorado, he decides to do a "walkthrough" of the trail on the day of his arrival. Starting at Leadville, he begins his methodical plodding along the route to the summit.

Critical Thinking Questions

1. What are some of the possible altitude sickness syndromes that would be suspected based on the mechanism of injury?

   _____

   _____

2. How does Jay's origin impact the chances of his contracting altitude sickness?

   _____

   _____

History

Halfway up the summit trail, Jay can no longer lift his legs. He is extremely short of breath and thinks he is going to pass out. A 60-year-old woman, Nellie, is walking the trail to the peak from her home near Leadville when she comes across Jay. "Are you all right, son?" she asks.

He explains, only getting out about one word at a time, that he is having trouble breathing. Nellie smiles, nods her head, and excuses herself for a moment to talk on the phone. "Hi, Jon?" she says. "It's Nellie. We got another flatlander on the trail. Send up the rescue team." Returning to Jay, she says, "Help is on the way. I am a Paramedic with the local search and rescue. Before they get here, maybe I can have a look at you."

Critical Thinking Questions

1. What are the important elements of the history that a Paramedic should obtain?

   _____

   _____

2. What questions should the Paramedic focus on in the medication history?

_____

_____

Examination

"Hey, Captain, look! He's Cheyne–Stokes breathing," the rookie says to Nellie. "Just get the oxygen on him," Nellie replies. "I'm trying," the rookie answers, "but he keeps coughing and ripping the mask off." Nellie looks up from Jay's fingers, which she notes are cyanotic, and says, "Jay, we need to get you off the mountain."

Critical Thinking Questions

1. What are the elements of the physical examination of a patient with suspected mountain sickness?

_____

_____

2. Why is a neurological examination a critical element in this examination?

_____

_____

Assessment

It seems to all add up. Jay is short of breath; he has dyspnea at rest; crackles are appreciated in one lung, but not the other; and he is cyanotic. Nellie checks off all the Lake Louise criteria to earn an admission at the regional medical center.

Critical Thinking Questions

1. What diagnosis did the Paramedic announce to the patient?

_____

_____

2. What other diagnosis is commonly associated with this diagnosis?

_____

_____

Treatment

"OK," says Nellie. "Change him over to the nasal cannula but keep his sat over 95%." "Should we start a line?" the rookie asks. "Maybe later," replies Nellie. "First, we need to get him off the mountain ASAP."

Critical Thinking Questions

1. What is the first priority for patients with suspected mountain sickness?

_____

_____

2. What are the priorities that follow?

_____

_____

Evaluation

"Hmm," Nellie mutters. "He doesn't seem to be getting much better yet. Let's call ahead and have them get the bag ready. Also, see if the helicopter can fly, please." Indeed, Jay's shortness of breath appears to be worsening and his oxygen saturation is dropping again.

Critical Thinking Questions

1. What are some treatments for advanced HAPE?

   _____

   _____

2. What is an experimental treatment that has shown promise in the treatment of advanced HAPE?

   _____

   _____

Disposition

The chopper from Airguard is spooling down as the crew arrives. Jay is sitting up in the back of the ambulance holding onto the oxygen mask for dear life. The crew gets a report from Nellie, thanks her, loads Jay into the chopper, and they are on their way. Jay looks out the helicopter window and sees the peak of Mt. Elbert as he flies by.

Critical Thinking Questions

1. What is the most appropriate transport decision that will get the patient to definitive care?

   _____

   _____

2. What are some of the transportation considerations?

   _____

   _____

Practice Questions
Multiple Choice

Select the best answer for each of the following questions.

1. Mt. McKinley, at over 20,000 feet, is the highest mountain in the United States. Its peak would be considered what type of altitude?
   a. high altitude
   b. extreme altitude
   c. severe altitude
   d. none of the above

2. Which law explains how the partial pressures at elevation can cause shortness of breath?
   a. Dalton's law
   b. Boyle's law
   c. Avogadro's law
   d. Henry's law

3. What is the first response to elevation?
   a. tachypnea
   b. polycythemia
   c. tachycardia
   d. hypertension

4. What is the respiratory pattern seen when a trekker sleeps?
   a. Cheyne–Stokes
   b. Kussmaul's
   c. hyperpnea
   d. Biot

5. Which of the following is NOT a risk factor for the development of high altitude cerebral edema?
   a. rapid ascent
   b. hyperventilation
   c. genes
   d. pulmonary disease

6. What causes high altitude pulmonary edema?
   a. hypervolemia
   b. increased pulmonary capillary pressure
   c. heart failure
   d. pulmonary capillary vasodilation

7. Which of the following is NOT a symptom of snow blindness?
   a. gritty feeling in the eyes
   b. pain with eyeball movement
   c. spots in the field of vision
   d. redness and tearing

8. Which of the following is NOT a symptom of high altitude pulmonary edema?
   a. extreme fatigue
   b. restlessness at night
   c. shortness of breath at rest
   d. hallucinations

9. What is the most common "first symptom" of mountain sickness?
   a. shortness of breath
   b. headache
   c. nausea
   d. coughing

10. What is the most effective treatment for high altitude cerebral edema?
    a. oxygen
    b. dexamethasone
    c. descent
    d. nifedipine

11. A Gamow bag is used for what condition?
    a. hypothermia
    b. HAPE
    c. HACE
    d. ASIA

12. What medication is useful to prepare a trekker?
    a. acetazolamide
    b. furosemide
    c. ibuprofen
    d. acetaminophen

13. What is the average "ceiling" for a helicopter?
    a. 5,000 meters
    b. 8,000 meters
    c. 10,000 meters
    d. 12,000 meters

14. What is the action of Diamox?
    a. acidifies blood
    b. diuresis
    c. anti-inflammatory
    d. analgesia

15. What is a common cause of headache at higher elevations?
    a. dehydration
    b. cerebral edema
    c. hypocapnia
    d. hypothermia

Short Answer

Write a brief answer to each of the following questions.

16. Describe acclimatization.

    _____

    _____

17. What are the body's three compensations for altitude-induced hypoxia?

    _____

    _____

18. Why does Cheyne–Stokes breathing occur?

    _____

    _____

19. How does one differentiate a headache from dehydration and a headache from HACE?

    _____

    _____

20. Why does high altitude retinal hemorrhage occur?

    _____

    _____

Fill in the Blank

Complete each sentence by adding the appropriate word in the provided blanks.

21. A dry persistent cough at higher elevations is called the _____ _____.

22. Ultraviolet keratitis is also called _____ _____.

23. The brand name for acetazolamide is _____.

24. The enzyme that lessens the affinity of oxygen to remain bound to hemoglobin is _____.

25. The process of physiologic adaption to altitude is called _____.

CHAPTER 15

WATER EMERGENCIES

Case Study

Chief Concern

"Coast Guard, do you copy? Dave just reported that Andre went unconscious while he was diving and, well, they made an emergency ascent. He will be topside in a moment. We need some help out here. Stand by, I am going to hit the emergency button on the DSC radio. That should give you our coordinates."

"Go ahead," the dispatcher replies as he alerts the closest Coast Guard cutter in the quadrant. The cutter *Confidence* steams toward the coordinates as shipboard medics prepare for the rescue mission.

Critical Thinking Questions

1. What are some of the possible causes of sudden unconsciousness while underwater?

   _____

   _____

2. What is the implication of an emergency ascent?

   _____

   _____

History

"He just popped out of the water like a rocket! Someone must have released his weight belt," the crew working topside reports. "He was complaining of having a headache and some double vision when suddenly he went limp." After this report is given to the Coast Guard medics, Andre is strapped to the litter for transfer to the cutter *Confidence*.

Critical Thinking Questions

1. What are the important elements of the history that a Paramedic should obtain?

   _____

   _____

2. What specific questions should the Paramedic ask, referring to the mechanism of injury?

   _____

   _____

Examination

The Coast Guard medic, Petty Officer Bloom, notes that the patient is unconscious as he lies in the litter but that he has a strong pulse, albeit a bradycardiac one, and he is hypertensive. Nothing else outwardly seems amiss.

"Let's get going!" Bloom yells out, as he makes a mental list of the things he will do when he gets back on deck of the cutter, "and keep that oxygen going. He needs it."

Critical Thinking Questions

1. What are the elements of the physical examination of a patient with suspected decompression sickness?

    _____

    _____

2. Why is a 12-lead ECG a critical element in this examination?

    _____

    _____

Assessment

"Captain, Petty Officer Bloom, sir. The patient is a 30-year-old male who is an inexperienced diver. Not sure what happened, but I think he may have rising intracranial pressure. He will need to be transferred stateside ASAP, sir."

Critical Thinking Questions

1. What diagnosis did the Paramedic announce to the crew?

    _____

    _____

2. What syndrome is suggested by the vital signs?

    _____

    _____

Treatment

The Coast Guard medic starts with a nasal airway and then applies high-flow, high-concentration oxygen via nonrebreather mask to the patient. Because no immediate treatment is anticipated, he delays establishing venous access until the patient is aboard the cutter *Confidence*.

Critical Thinking Questions

1. What is the national standard of care of patients with suspected decompression sickness, specifically cerebral arterial gas embolism?

    _____

    _____

2. What can be done if venous access is not readily obtainable?

    _____

    _____

Evaluation

"Hi Doc, he's breathing funny." Medic Bloom looks down and notes the asymmetrical rise and fall of the patient's chest. "He must have a pneumothorax. What's his blood pressure now?" he asks as he assesses the throat for tracheal tugging and looks for jugular venous distention.

Critical Thinking Questions

1. What are some of the predictable complications associated with an emergency ascent?

    _____

    _____

2. What are some of the concerns for a drowned diver?

_____

_____

Disposition

Safely aboard the H-65 *Dolphin*, Andre is flown to the regional trauma center some 65 nautical miles south of the cutter *Confidence*. As he is attended to by two experienced Coast Guard medics, Petty Officer Bloom knows Andre has the best chance for survival.

Critical Thinking Questions

1. What is the most appropriate transport decision that will get the patient to definitive care?

_____

_____

2. What is the optimal transportation decision?

_____

_____

Practice Questions

Multiple Choice

Select the best answer for each of the following questions.

1. Dry drownings make up what percentage of all drownings?
   a. 70%
   b. 50%
   c. 30%
   d. 10%

2. What is the "thermoneutral" point of water temperature?
   a. 70°F
   b. 77°F
   c. 80°F
   d. 91°F

3. Which gas law states the greater the pressure, the smaller the volume?
   a. Boyle's law
   b. Dalton's law
   c. Henry's law
   d. Charles' law

4. Which gas law states the partial pressure of a gas increases as the pressure of the whole gas increases?
   a. Boyle's law
   b. Dalton's law
   c. Henry's law
   d. Charles' law

5. Which gas law states the amount of gas dissolved in liquid is proportional to the partial pressure of that gas?
   a. Boyle's law
   b. Dalton's law
   c. Henry's law
   d. Charles' law

6. Which gas law states the colder the water, the more the pressure decreases?
   a. Boyle's law
   b. Dalton's law
   c. Henry's law
   d. Charles' law

7. "Executive functions" are affected by what condition?
   a. nitrogen narcosis
   b. the bends
   c. immersion pulmonary edema
   d. the chokes

8. What is the appearance of nitrogen under the skin that makes the skin feel like it is crawling called?
   a. cutis marmorata
   b. formication
   c. subcutaneous emphysema
   d. chokes

9. Which of the following is NOT associated with decompression sickness?
   a. formication
   b. ascending paralysis
   c. burning chest pain
   d. hallucinations

10. Which of the following is NOT associated with the "chokes"?
    a. dry hacking cough
    b. pleuritic chest pain
    c. hypoxia
    d. fulminate pulmonary edema

11. Which hyperbaric condition can mimic a stroke?
    a. cerebral arterial gas embolism
    b. immersion pulmonary edema
    c. pulmonary decompression sickness
    d. pulmonary barotrauma

12. The patient with which of the following conditions is NOT prone to barotrauma?
    a. history of COPD
    b. bronchitis
    c. history of pulmonary cysts
    d. lung cancer

13. Which of the following is NOT a minor dive syndrome?
    a. sinus squeeze
    b. ear squeeze
    c. eye squeeze
    d. tooth squeeze

14. Which of the following is NOT a symptom of decompression sickness I (DCS I)?
    a. headache
    b. skin symptoms
    c. musculoskeletal pain
    d. stomach pain

15. Which of the following is NOT a symptom of decompression sickness II (DCS II)?
    a. double vision
    b. lower back pain
    c. joint pain
    d. ascending paralysis

Short Answer

Write a brief answer to each of the following questions.

16. Why would a floating body possibly indicate murder instead of drowning?

    _____

    _____

17. What is the problem with a patent foramen ovale and divers?

    _____

    _____

18. Differentiate the U.S. Navy classifications of decompression sickness I and decompression sickness II.

    _____

    _____

19. List the symptom pattern of decompression sickness.

    _____

    _____

20. What occurs during a panic ascent?

    _____

    _____

Fill in the Blank

Complete each sentence by adding the appropriate word in the provided blanks.

21. Hyperventilation before snorkeling leads to _____ _____ _____.

22. Rapture of the deep is also called _____ _____.

23. The other name for pulmonary decompression sickness is the _____.

24. A spot in the eyes, due to decompression sickness, is called _____.

25. A rash, secondary to decompression, that leaves the skin marbled in appearance is called _____ _____.

CHAPTER 16

ENVENOMATION

Case Study

Chief Concern

"Just another day in paradise," Dan sighs. He has been assigned to the coveted beach duty, which means he gets to drive up and down the beach, enjoying the fresh air and sunshine.

Dan's moment of nirvana is interrupted by a middle-aged woman who is running toward him. She yells that her husband has been bitten by a jellyfish.

Critical Thinking Questions

1. What are some of the possible venomous marine life forms that a swimmer could encounter?

   _____

   _____

2. Which of these marine life forms is not a jellyfish?

   _____

   _____

History

The older gentleman explains that he had been swimming when he spotted a Portuguese man-o-war. He heard that they had been swarming and wanted to get a look. He thought he kept his distance, about 10 yards, when he felt something painful on his ankle and realized he had been ensnared in a tentacle.

The pain was excruciating, and a helpful bystander told him to urinate on his leg. The only thing that did was make him feel ridiculous. The pain became much worse, so bad that he started yelling. His wife immediately left him to get help.

Critical Thinking Questions

1. What are the important elements of the history that a Paramedic should obtain?

   _____

   _____

2. What is the symptom pattern associated with a Portuguese man-o-war jellyfish bite?

   _____

   _____

Examination

Dan begins a standard examination. The patient is grasping his ankle, which looks red and angry. Remembering what he has been told about the patient urinating on his leg, Dan puts on his gloves to get a closer look.

Dan sees multiple whip-like welts and a papular rash along the welt. Carefully, Dan starts to pick up the visible tentacles with his gloved hand. Next, he takes a child's sand pail, fills it with water from the ocean, and pours it over the patient's legs.

Critical Thinking Questions

1. What are the elements of the physical examination of a patient with a suspected jellyfish sting?

_____

_____

2. What other reactions might occur as a result of the envenomation?

_____

_____

Assessment

"Yep," Dan says. "You certainly got stung by a man-o-war. Fortunately, there is something I can do to help you. Do you have an ice cold beer in that chest?" Both the wife and the patient look at Dan quizzically.

Critical Thinking Questions

1. What diagnosis did the Paramedic announce to the patient?

_____

_____

2. What secondary diagnosis might be associated with the primary diagnosis?

_____

_____

Treatment

"Well, specifically I need the ice," Dan explains. The wife returns shortly with a plastic bag filled with ice. The patient's relief from the ice is almost immediate!

Critical Thinking Questions

1. What is the national standard of care of patients with suspected marine envenomation?

_____

_____

2. What are some of the patient-specific concerns and considerations that the Paramedic should consider when applying this plan of care for patients presenting with suspected marine envenomation?

_____

_____

Evaluation

Dan continues his assessment. "Are you sure that he didn't hit you anywhere else? The pain in your leg can be distracting. He didn't sting your face or eyes?"

The patient denies any further injury but complains his leg still hurts. "Well, let me give you some Benadryl and let's get you back to the camper for a hot shower, and I mean hot!" Dan explains.

Critical Thinking Questions

1. What are some of the predictable complications associated with a sting from the Portuguese man-o-war?

   _____

   _____

2. What is the treatment to prevent these complications?

   _____

   _____

Disposition

"Seriously, I can't let you drive after giving you that Benadryl," Dan states. "Benadryl makes you sleepy and I don't want to have to treat you for trauma as well. Please take advantage of the ambulance and go to the local hospital."

Critical Thinking Questions

1. What is the most appropriate transport decision that will get the patient to definitive care?

   _____

   _____

2. What if the patient refuses further care or transport?

   _____

   _____

Practice Questions

Multiple Choice

Select the best answer for each of the following questions.

1. Which of the following is NOT part of the order Hymenoptera?
   a. bees
   b. wasps
   c. ants
   d. termites

2. In which of the following states do venomous snakes exist?
   a. Alaska
   b. Hawaii
   c. North Dakota
   d. Maine

3. What family is responsible for the majority of poisonous snake envenomations?
   a. Viperidae
   b. Elapidae
   c. Colubridae
   d. Formicidae

4. Which of the following snakes is NOT in the family Viperidae Crotalinae?
   a. rattlesnakes
   b. coral snakes
   c. cottonmouth
   d. copperhead

5. Which of the following is NOT a characteristic of venomous snakes?
   a. fangs
   b. double row of scales
   c. elliptical pupils
   d. sensory pits

6. The characteristic hourglass shape on the ventral surface is only found on the _____ species.
   a. *L. mactans* (black widow)
   b. *L. hesperus* (western black widow)
   c. *L. bishopi* (brown widow)
   d. *L. geometricus* (brown button widow)

7. A black widow spider's venom contains _____.
   a. hemolysin
   b. alpha-latrotoxin
   c. formic acid
   d. hyaluronidase

8. Brown recluse spider venom contains _____.
   a. hemolysin
   b. alpha–latrotoxin
   c. formic acid
   d. hylaurinadase

9. Scorpion venom is primarily _____.
   a. neurotoxic
   b. cytotoxic
   c. hemolytic
   d. nephrotoxic

10. Which of the following is responsible for the most fatalities attributed to venomous marine life?
    a. man-o-war
    b. fire coral
    c. sea nettle
    d. Hawaiian box jellyfish

11. Which of the following is NOT a jellyfish?
    a. Hydrozoa
    b. Cubozoa
    c. Anthozoa
    d. Scyphozoa

12. Which of the following will NOT occur with a hymenoptera bite?
    a. swelling
    b. necrosis
    c. erythema
    d. pruritus

13. Which of the following is NOT a sign of an anaphylactic reaction?
    a. erythema
    b. urticaria
    c. pruritus
    d. angioedema

14. How many fang marks can appear from a snakebite?
    a. one fang mark
    b. two fang marks
    c. no fang marks
    d. all of the above

15. Which of the following produces a halo around the bite site, as well as localized piloerection with hidrosis?
    a. black widow spider bite
    b. yellow jacket sting
    c. rattlesnake bite
    d. Africanized bee sting

Short Answer

Write a brief answer to each of the following questions.

16. What is the mechanism of action for the black widow spider venom?

    _____

    _____

17. What is the mechanism of action for the scorpion bite?

    _____

    _____

18. Why should tourniquets be avoided for snake bites?

    _____

    _____

19. What is the treatment for a jellyfish bite?

    _____

    _____

20. What is seabather's eruption?

    _____

    _____

Fill in the Blank

Complete each sentence by adding the appropriate word in the provided blanks.

21. Ants bite and spray venom that includes formic acid and _____, a chemical that breaks down red blood cells.

22. Perhaps the most notable distinguishing characteristic of a pit viper is its _____ head.

23. "Red on yellow, kill a fellow; red on black, friend of Jack" is a rhyme that refers to the _____ snake.

24. An unusual pattern of facial swelling accompanied by ptosis and rhinitis is called _____ _____.

25. The lesion from a recluse spider bite is called _____ _____.

CHAPTER 17

EMS VEHICLE AND TRANSPORT SAFETY

Case Study

"Not quite sure why I got this assignment, Captain," Tony says.

"Well, rookie," the captain replies. "As the new guy here, we thought you might bring a fresh perspective to the topic. We only spec out ambulances every five years. I'll be retiring next year and, well, you won't. Since you'll have to put up with the monster that we create, it only seems right that you should pick your own poison!"

After hearing those words, Tony decides he is going to research the daylights out of ambulance safety.

Critical Thinking Questions

1. What are the vehicle safety standards for ambulance construction?

_____

_____

2. What can be done to make the patient compartment safer for all of the occupants?

_____

_____

"Well," says the captain, inspecting the ambulance design, "We have quite a camel here!" Based on Tony's quizzical expression, the captain explains how he's referring to the joke about the committee that was charged to design a horse for the desert and created a camel. "This is quite a departure from the past, but hey, at least I don't have to live with it." Despite the captain's chuckles, Tony is proud of the new ambulance design.

Critical Thinking Questions

3. What safety performance modifications to an ambulance will increase its crashworthiness?

_____

_____

4. What liability does the service hold if this ambulance is involved in a crash? What is the likelihood that the service will be sued?

_____

_____

Practice Questions

Multiple Choice

Select the best answer for each of the following questions.

1. Which federal initiative is expected to have a positive impact on EMS safety while providers are on scene?
   a. Worker Visibility Act
   b. Highway Renewal Act
   c. Highway Safety Act
   d. NFPA PPE Act

2. Which of the following was NOT identified as an inexpensive safety engineering item for ambulances that can be immediately implemented?
   a. oxygen cylinders stored in soft cases
   b. over-the-shoulder harnesses on a gurney
   c. seat belt use in the patient compartment
   d. secured equipment in the patient compartment

3. What is the highest-risk driving practice when operating an ambulance?
   a. failing to use the siren with lights
   b. failing to pass on the left side
   c. failing to drive at the posted speed limit
   d. failing to stop at a red light

4. Which of the following is the only nationally approved safety standard for ambulances?
   a. National Fire Protection Association Standard 314
   b. Federal Highway Safety Standard KKK–2222
   c. American Ambulance Association Standard 34-1
   d. American Society of Safety Engineers Z15.1 Fleet Safety Standard

5. Which of the following provides real-time driver monitoring?
   a. intelligent transportation systems
   b. in-vehicle telematics technology
   c. iron sergeant driver safety monitors
   d. OnStar® vehicle safety monitoring

6. What is the only expert panel-derived risk and safety awareness driver training course?
   a. Ambulance Accident Course
   b. Emergency Vehicle Operators Course
   c. National Ambulance Drivers Course
   d. EMS Safety Course

7. Which of the following is the preferred seating arrangement in the patient compartment of an ambulance?
   a. rear-facing captain's chair
   b. seat-belted on bench seat
   c. forward-facing bucket seats
   d. pedestal style seating

8. What is the most dangerous type of harness?
   a. trapeze harness
   b. lap belt
   c. three-point harness
   d. harness restraint system

9. According to one study, over three-quarters of ambulance crashes are caused by _____.
   a. a small number of unsafe drivers
   b. unsafe stopping
   c. brake failure
   d. failure to use both lights and siren

10. What causes over three-quarters of fatalities in ambulance collisons?
    a. unbelted providers
    b. flying equipment
    c. unpadded compartments
    d. collisions with patients

11. Which of the following is responsible for one in five EMS provider deaths in the line of duty?
    a. being struck by a passing motorist
    b. being in an ambulance rollover
    c. being thrown in a patient compartment
    d. being in an intersection collision

12. Which of the following is NOT a hazard that has been identified in ambulance compartments?
    a. blunt head strike zones
    b. noncrashworthy patient compartment
    c. lack of crumple zones
    d. over-the-shoulder patient harness

13. What are the most hazardous vehicles on the road?
    a. passenger cars
    b. trucks
    c. police cruisers
    d. ambulances

14. The duration of a crash is comparable to what amount of time?
    a. the time it takes to read this answer
    b. the time it takes to put on a seat belt
    c. the time it takes to blink one's eye
    d. the time it takes to sit down

15. Which of the following air medical practices should ambulances NOT consider putting into practice?
    a. preflight safety checklists
    b. protective helmets
    c. pilot–crew communications
    d. mission clearance

Short Answer

Write a brief answer to each of the following questions.

16. What are some of the attributes to consider when designing head protection for EMS providers?

    _____

    _____

17. What are the optimal colors Paramedics should wear during the day and night?

    _____

    _____

18. What does the National Institute of Occupational Safety and Health (NIOSH) do?

_____

_____

19. What danger do Paramedics face by wearing dark blue uniforms or even fluorescent vests on scene at night?

_____

_____

20. What is in-vehicle telematics technology?

_____

_____

Fill in the Blank

Complete each sentence by adding the appropriate word in the provided blanks.

21. Ambulances are largely exempt from the _____ _____ _____ _____ Standards.

22. The _____ visibility reflective markings, which are popular in Europe, have largely fallen out of favor in the United States.

23. A _____ would prevent head injuries during ambulance collisions.

24. The _____ _____ Act ensures that EMS providers wear reflective protective clothing while on scene at a road emergency.

25. The _____ specifications of the federal General Services Administration only provide purchase specifications, not safety performance standards.

CHAPTER 18

AIR MEDICAL TRANSPORT

Case Study

The team is just starting to set up ropes for the descent. It seems that two hikers have slipped over the edge of the falls and are now at the bottom of a steep ravine. "Better call the chopper!" the team leader cries out to the operations officer. "This is going to take some time!"

Critical Thinking Questions

1. What are some of the possible advantages of helicopter transport?

   _____

   _____

2. What conditions warrant air medical service?

   _____

   _____

With the helicopter safely lifted off and on its way, the landing zone crew prepares to lounge for 20 minutes. It is company policy to keep the LZ open for 20 minutes in case an emergency landing is needed.

   While picking up the cones that marked the landing zone, the firefighters comment on the incredible luck of the two hikers. Several factors—making a call on a GPS-capable cell phone, being rescued by an ever-ready local rope team, and having an air medical service available—optimized their chance of survival.

Critical Thinking Questions

3. What is the most appropriate transport decision that will get the patient to definitive care?

   _____

   _____

4. What are the advantages of transporting a patient with suspected trauma to these hospitals, even if that means bypassing other hospitals in the process?

   _____

   _____

Practice Questions

Multiple Choice

Select the best answer for each of the following questions.

1. What was the first large-scale conflict during which helicopters were used for air medical evacuation?
   a. World War I
   b. World War II
   c. Korea
   d. Vietnam

2. What was the first civilian air medical unit?
   a. St. Anthony's Hospital
   b. LifeNet
   c. Maryland state police
   d. Military Assistance to Safety and Traffic (MAST)

3. Which of the following is the standard flight crew configuration?
   a. Paramedic/nurse
   b. Paramedic/Paramedic
   c. Paramedic/respiratory therapist
   d. Paramedic/physician

4. Which of the following members of the air medical crew typically needs additional training in advanced airway management?
   a. nurse
   b. Paramedic
   c. physician
   d. respiratory therapist

5. Which of the following is least likely to be a member of the flight crew?
   a. nurse
   b. Paramedic
   c. physician
   d. respiratory therapist

6. What group has put forth "Guidelines of Air Medical Dispatch"?
   a. Emergency Dispatch Association
   b. Emergency Medical Dispatch
   c. National Association of Flight Paramedics
   d. National Association of EMS Physicians

7. Failure to use a helicopter when indicated is an example of _____.
   a. undertriage
   b. underutilization
   c. undercriticality
   d. overtriage

8. Which of the following is NOT part of the auto-launch criteria established by the Association of Air Medical Services?
   a. long flight distance (>29 miles)
   b. multiple casualty incident
   c. critical burns
   d. acute myocardial infarction

9. Which of the following is NOT considered a time-sensitive condition?
   a. stroke
   b. acute myocardial infarction
   c. severe trauma
   d. trauma arrest without return of spontaneous circulation

10. Which of the following dictates requirements for interfacility transfers?
    a. National Association of EMS Physicians
    b. Emergency Medical Treatment and Active Labor Act
    c. Consolidated Omnibus Budget Reconciliation Act
    d. local hospital protocol

11. Which law of gasses probably has the greatest impact on flight physiology?
    a. Dalton's law
    b. Boyle's law
    c. Avogadro's law
    d. Curtis's law

12. Which of the following is NOT an area where gasses can expand?
    a. teeth
    b. sinus
    c. lungs
    d. bladder

13. What factor that leads to fatigue is somewhat unique to the air medical service?
    a. inadequate sleep
    b. dehydration
    c. vibration
    d. poor diet

14. What is the preferred size of the touchdown zone for a helicopter?
    a. 50 × 50 feet
    b. 50 × 75 feet
    c. 75 × 100 feet
    d. 100 × 100 feet

15. What presents the greatest danger to a helicopter when landing?
    a. trees
    b. flares
    c. buildings
    d. telephone wires

Short Answer

Write a brief answer to each of the following questions.

16. What can be used to mark a landing zone?

   _____

   _____

17. Why should a Paramedic wear a safety helmet in the landing zone?

   _____

   _____

18. How should a Paramedic approach a helicopter?

_____

_____

19. What is the "culture of safety"?

_____

_____

20. What organization accredits air medical services?

_____

_____

Fill in the Blank

Complete each sentence by adding the appropriate word in the provided blanks.

21. Simultaneous dispatch of a helicopter and local ground ambulances at the time of dispatch is part of a _____ _____ policy.

22. Debris stirred up by the helicopter is called _____ _____.

23. Vigorous crossing and uncrossing of the hands over the head is called the _____ _____.

24. A helicopter that does not shut down for loading, in which the rotors remain spinning, is referred to as a _____ _____.

25. Helicopters are also referred to as _____ _____ aircraft.

CHAPTER 19

SPECIALTY CARE TRANSPORT

Case Study

Seth is on call for the pediatric specialty care transport unit, and just as he is about to sit down for dinner his pager goes off. He sighs at the interruption, although he remembers that the on-call pay, as well as a special care transport bonus on top of his regular pay, make these interruptions a little more bearable.

The team members—consisting of a driver, a Paramedic, and Seth—simultaneously arrive in the emergency department and await the arriving ambulance. The patient, a small boy who was hit by a car, survived the initial impact. However, he ruptured his spleen, lacerated his liver, and punctured his lung. As the ambulance pulls into the emergency department bay, the team is greeted by the gentle sound of the air moving up and down the patient's ventilator circuit.

Critical Thinking Questions

1. What are some of the possible complications that the Paramedic may encounter en route to the receiving hospital?

   _____

   _____

2. What is the "problem list" that the Paramedic must monitor?

   _____

   _____

Seth and his crew quickly transport the boy to the regional trauma center. Upon their arrival, Seth gives report to the receiving physician. Although Seth has authority to start vasopressors as needed, as outlined in the patient care guidelines and the transferring facility's medical orders, they are not needed, as the patient has remained stable throughout the trip.

The little boy, still paralyzed and on a ventilator, is immediately transferred to the pediatric intensive care unit by Seth and his team.

Critical Thinking Questions

3. What is the most appropriate transport decision that will get the patient to definitive care?

   _____

   _____

4. What are the advantages of transporting a patient with suspected spinal cord injury to these hospitals, even if that means bypassing other hospitals in the process?

   _____

   _____

Practice Questions

Multiple Choice

Select the best answer for each of the following questions.

1. Which of the following is NOT a currently accepted specialty hospital?
   a. trauma
   b. stroke
   c. STEMI
   d. organ transplant

2. The Emergency Medical Treatment and Active Labor Act was specifically passed to prevent denial of treatment because of what reason?
   a. inability to pay
   b. race
   c. ethnicity
   d. country of origin

3. EMTALA speaks to hospital destination specifically for which type of EMS?
   a. fire-based EMS
   b. private commercial EMS
   c. hospital-based EMS
   d. volunteer EMS

4. Which of the following requirements must be met before transferring a patient?
   a. medical necessity
   b. ability to pay
   c. acceptance of transfer
   d. adequate ambulance service

5. Which of the following does NOT need to be arranged before the patient can be transferred?
   a. acceptance of patient for transfer
   b. transfer of pertinent medical documentation
   c. arrangements for family to stay near accepting facility
   d. qualified personnel used during transfer

6. Which of the following is NOT taken into consideration when defining the ambulance's crew configuration?
   a. patient's illness
   b. complexity of illness
   c. insurance coverage
   d. frequency of assessments

7. Which of the following medical devices is NOT typically transported by a traditional Paramedic?
   a. thoracostomy drainage tube
   b. indwelling urinary catheter
   c. non-medicated intravenous infusion
   d. advanced mechanical ventilation

8. Which of the following may be transported by a traditional Paramedic?
   a. ventriculostomy requiring maintenance
   b. transvenous pacer requiring maintenance
   c. parenteral bolus medication
   d. left ventricular assist device

9. Which of the following topics is not covered in a Paramedic's original education?
   a. infectious diseases
   b. ventilator management
   c. hemodynamic monitoring
   d. biomedical devices

10. Which of the following common conditions does NOT require an interfacility transfer to a specialty hospital?
    a. traumatic brain injury
    b. high-risk obstetrics
    c. orthopedic injury
    d. spinal cord injury

11. Which of the following statements is true about the chest tube?
    a. It should never be dependent for drainage.
    b. It should never be clamped during transfer.
    c. It should not be on intermittent suction.
    d. It should not be turned on its side.

12. Which of the following is NOT considered central line venous access?
    a. femoral line
    b. internal jugular line
    c. subclavian line
    d. external jugular line

13. The pulmonary artery catheter does NOT allow measurement of which of the following values?
    a. central venous pressure
    b. pulmonary artery pressure
    c. cardiac output
    d. pulmonary capillary wedge pressure

14. If a patient is bleeding from a noncompressible site and is on Coumadin, which of the following blood products may be transfused?
    a. fresh frozen plasma
    b. packed red blood cells
    c. whole blood
    d. plasmapheresis

15. Which of the following blood transfusion reactions occurs in less than 15 minutes?
    a. febrile
    b. allergic
    c. septic
    d. hemolytic

Short Answer

Write a brief answer to each of the following questions.

16. Define specialization of hospitals.

_____

_____

17. Define reverse dumping.

_____

_____

18. What is the EMTALA definition of an unstable patient?

_____

_____

19. What indicates a Paramedic with training for specialty care transport?

_____

_____

20. What differentiates protocols from patient care guidelines?

_____

_____

Fill in the Blank

Complete each sentence by adding the appropriate word in the provided blanks.

21. A higher level of reimbursement allowed by the Centers for Medicare and Medicaid for complex patients is called _____ _____ _____.

22. Reaction to blood in which the patient's blood is incompatible with the transfusion is called a _____ _____.

23. In 1985, Congress enacted a law that was intended to prevent unethical practice called the _____ _____ _____ and _____ _____ _____.

24. Paramedics receive a set of orders for interfacility transfers called _____ _____ _____.

25. A transducer is leveled to the _____ _____.

CHAPTER 20

NATIONAL INCIDENT MANAGEMENT SYSTEM

Case Study

The flooding is massive. The river hit the century mark, moved well past flood stage, and breeched the levies. Despite the best efforts of the local residents, the water continues to flood the streets. Many people have already been evacuated, although a few holdouts remain who never thought the river would get so high. The drone of a helicopter, carrying the governor, can be heard overhead.

Looking out the helicopter's window, she quietly says, "Oh my god. Order out the National Guard and get me connected to the federal folks!"

Critical Thinking Questions

1. What is the National Response Framework for a mass-casualty incident?

   _____

   _____

2. What law empowers the federal government to activate reservists and disaster teams, as well as call for volunteers?

   _____

   _____

The crews are happy to see the National Guardsmen roll up in those "deuce and a half" trucks loaded with supplies from the Strategic National Stockpile. Although all of the roads into the area are flooded, the Guard is able to airlift supplies to the drop point.

Accompanying the Guardsmen are members of the Medical Reserve Corps. These medical providers are a welcome sight to the beleaguered doctors and nurses who have been providing around-the-clock care for the last 48 hours.

Critical Thinking Questions

3. What is the Strategic National Stockpile?

   _____

   _____

4. What is the Medical Reserve Corps?

   _____

   _____

Practice Questions

Multiple Choice

Select the best answer for each of the following questions.

1. Which of the following authorities is NOT considered essential to the federal emergency response?
   a. Stafford Disaster Relief Act
   b. Homeland Security Act
   c. Post-Katrina Emergency Management Reform Act
   d. Health and Human Services Act

2. Which act defines the provisions for federal disaster relief?
   a. Stafford Disaster Relief Act
   b. Homeland Security Act
   c. Post-Katrina Emergency Management Reform Act
   d. Health and Human Services Act

3. Which act clarifies the responsibilities of the federal government during a disaster?
   a. Stafford Disaster Relief Act
   b. Homeland Security Act
   c. Post-Katrina Emergency Management Reform Act
   d. Health and Human Services Act

4. What law/act or presidential directive requires an "all-hazards" approach to disaster preparedness?
   a. National Response Plan
   b. Homeland Security Directive
   c. Stafford Act
   d. Homeland Security Act

5. Which of the following is NOT a scenario in the National Preparedness Guidelines?
   a. plague
   b. cyber attack
   c. food contamination
   d. assassination

6. Who is the federal official with overall authority of a disaster?
   a. secretary of homeland security
   b. attorney general
   c. secretary of defense
   d. president

7. The attorney general uses the _____ to investigate terrorism.
   a. Federal Bureau of Investigation
   b. Central Intelligence Agency
   c. Federal Bureau of Firearms, Alcohol, and Tobacco
   d. Naval Criminal Investigation Service

8. What group is responsible for overall situational awareness in a disaster?
   a. National Operations Center
   b. Homeland Security Information Network
   c. Department of Health and Human Services
   d. National Disaster Management System

9. Paramedics typically are NOT involved in which of the following Emergency Support Functions?
   a. Firefighting (4)
   b. Emergency Management (5)
   c. Mass Care and Housing (6)
   d. Urban Search and Rescue (9)

10. Which location features the highest level of command and control?
    a. Joint Field Office
    b. Incident Command Post
    c. Area Wide Command
    d. Local Emergency Operations Center

11. Which group does NOT manage on-scene operations?
    a. Joint Field Office
    b. Incident Command Post
    c. Area Wide Command
    d. Local Emergency Operations Center

12. Which of the following individuals is NOT a member of the Joint Field Office staff?
    a. safety officer
    b. legal affairs advisor
    c. defense coordinating officer
    d. incident commander

13. Which of the following individuals is NOT a member of the Command Post staff?
    a. information officer
    b. liaison officer
    c. safety officer
    d. legal affairs officer

14. Which of the following is NOT part of the National Incident Management System?
    a. preparedness
    b. communications and information management
    c. command and management
    d. mitigation

15. Mutual aid agreements are part of the _____ component of the National Incident Management System.
    a. preparedness
    b. communications and information management
    c. command and management
    d. mitigation

Short Answer

Write a brief answer to each of the following questions.

16. What act prevents an area from using the military in a law enforcement capacity?

_____

_____

17. Name three specialty disaster response teams.

_____

_____

18. What is the purpose of the Strategic National Stockpile?

_____

_____

19. What is a CHEMPACK?

_____

_____

20. How are civilian volunteers integrated into the National Incident Management System?

_____

_____

Fill in the Blank

Complete each sentence by adding the appropriate word in the provided blanks.

21. The Federal Response Plan evolved, following the 9/11 terrorist attacks, into the _____ _____ _____.

22. Members of the media get their information regarding an incident from the _____ _____ _____.

23. Supporting federal communications is the _____ _____ and _____ _____ detachment.

24. The _____ _____ _____ _____ task force is called in the event of an earthquake.

25. Volunteer healthcare providers are part of the _____ _____ _____ _____.

CHAPTER **21**

EMERGENCY RESPONSE TO TERRORISM

Case Study

"Hmm," Shelley murmurs. "This is the fifth patient we have picked up today with severe cold symptoms and all are from the same neighborhood." Shelley wonders if this may be more than a coincidence, as she remembers her recent terrorism lecture. The terrorism lectures were mandatory for all responders after local law enforcement had received a credible threat warning of terrorist activity.

Critical Thinking Questions

1. What is the implication of multiple patients with the same symptoms?

_____

_____

2. What protection should the Paramedic take against these forms of terrorism?

_____

_____

By the end of the day, several "sick person" calls had blossomed into several hundred calls and the city's hospitals were brimming over. His honor the mayor, in an address covered by both public radio and television, instructs the public to stay home, telling them aid will come to them. In short, the mayor institutes a quarantine.

Critical Thinking Questions

3. What is the preferred response to a terrorist threat?

_____

_____

4. Why would terrorists use an infectious agent as the weapon of choice?

_____

_____

Practice Questions

Multiple Choice

Select the best answer for each of the following questions.

1. A white supremacist would be considered part of which group?
   a. right-wing extremists
   b. special interest groups
   c. left-wing extremists
   d. foreign terrorists

2. Which of the following terms does NOT describe left-wing extremists?
   a. anticapitalists
   b. antigovernment
   c. racist
   d. antiregulation

3. Which of the following is NOT considered a special interest group?
   a. anti-fur groups
   b. animal rights group
   c. environmentalists
   d. religious extremists

4. Which of the following groups may pose the greatest terrorist threat?
   a. right-wing extremists
   b. lone wolf terrorists
   c. white supremacists
   d. animal rights groups

5. The date April 19 is significant to which of the following groups?
   a. right-wing extremists
   b. lone wolf terrorists
   c. white supremacists
   d. animal rights groups

6. The date April 20 is the anniversary of which terrorist-related event?
   a. Waco
   b. Oklahoma City
   c. Ruby Ridge
   d. Columbine

7. Which of the following does NOT limit the Paramedic's exposure to weapons of mass destruction?
   a. time
   b. distance
   c. decontamination
   d. shielding

8. Which of the following is NOT a "blood poison"?
   a. hydrogen cyanide
   b. phosgene
   c. carbon monoxide
   d. ethylene

9. Which of the following is NOT a simple asphyxiant, a gas that is "inert" and simply displaces oxygen?
   a. carbon monoxide
   b. hydrogen
   c. carbon dioxide
   d. propane

10. Which of the following is NOT eliminated by antibiotics?
    a. *Bacillus anthracis*
    b. *Yersinia pestis*
    c. *Variola major*
    d. *Francisella tularensis*

11. Which of the following bacteria is NOT contagious?
    a. *Clostridium botulinum*
    b. *Francisella tularensis*
    c. *Yersinia pestis*
    d. *Bacillus anthracis*

12. Which of the following is a form of armed attack?
    a. assassination
    b. hostage taking
    c. hijacking
    d. all of the above

13. Which of the following is NOT a mnemonic to help providers remember forms of harm caused by terrorism?
    a. TRACEM
    b. TERORS
    c. CBRNE
    d. B-NICE

14. Which of the following is NOT a living organism?
    a. botulism
    b. Francisella tularensis
    c. Yersinia pestis
    d. Bacillus anthracis

15. What is the next form of terrorism expected in the United States?
    a. cyberterrorism
    b. assassination
    c. hijacking
    d. suicide bomber

Short Answer

Write a brief answer to each of the following questions.

16. Define terrorism.

_____

_____

17. What are the core principles of right-wing extremists?

_____

_____

18. What are the core principles of left-wing extremists?

_____

_____

19. What is the mnemonic for the symptom pattern associated with organophosphate poisoning?

_____

_____

20. What are blood agents?

_____

_____

Fill in the Blank

Complete each sentence by adding the appropriate word in the provided blanks.

21. Being ever vigilant of attack on scene is called _____ _____.

22. A pattern of illness or similar symptoms is called a _____.

23. A bomb that contains nuclear materials for dispersal during explosion is called a _____
_____.

24. The antidote for organophosphate poisoning is atropine and _____ _____ (2-PAM).

25. Explosive devices meant to harm responders are called _____ _____.

CHAPTER 22

PUBLIC HEALTH EMERGENCY PREPAREDNESS AND RESPONSE

Case Study

The city decides to use the scenario of a contaminated water supply for its drill. The story goes that terrorists seeded a local water supply with a poison and have created a public panic. The Paramedics of the Able Ambulance Association have been asked to perform triage. "Where do we set up?" the rookie asks.

Critical Thinking Questions

1. How does triage differ in a public health emergency?

   _____

   _____

2. What are some techniques used to prevent the spread of an infectious disease?

   _____

   _____

Several Paramedics have been ordered to the "POD" to assist the county health nurses. Incident Command is starting to feel the strain of responding to its many requests for help with only its limited pool of personnel. In fact, in response to one request for help, IC issues instructions to send one-and-a-half Paramedics.

The crew chief laughs at the impossible request. "Does he mean send an EMT and a Paramedic, or do one of you want to go and ask for clarification?"

Critical Thinking Questions

3. What "out of scope of practice" duties might a Paramedic perform in this situation?

   _____

   _____

4. What training could Paramedics perform that would prepare them for these roles?

   _____

   _____

Practice Questions

Multiple Choice

Select the best answer for each of the following questions.

1. Which of the following terms does NOT describe a public health emergency?
   a. micro-events
   b. poorly demarcated
   c. confined
   d. escalating

2. Which of the following is NOT an example of a public health emergency?
   a. food-borne illness outbreak
   b. multi-vehicle collision
   c. bioterrorism
   d. chemical release

3. What might be the greatest danger in a public health emergency?
   a. public panic
   b. scarcity of medical supplies
   c. poorly trained personnel
   d. poor preplanning

4. Which of the following is NOT a core principle of public health?
   a. prevent
   b. isolate
   c. mitigate
   d. treat

5. What would likely change for the Paramedic during a public health emergency?
   a. mode of transportation
   b. means of care
   c. scope of practice
   d. medical command

6. What term describes the separation of infected individuals to prevent the spread of disease?
   a. isolation
   b. protect in place
   c. social distancing
   d. ring vaccination

7. What term describes the suspension of normal activities to prevent unnecessary person-to-person contact in hopes of preventing transmission of infection?
   a. isolation
   b. protect in place
   c. social distancing
   d. ring vaccination

8. What term describes the prevention of the spread of infection by special immunization to a large number of people?
   a. isolation
   b. protect in place
   c. social distancing
   d. ring vaccination

9. Which of the following situations will NOT be prevented by cooperation and preplanning?
   a. inadequate personnel
   b. scarcity of medical supplies
   c. communications difficulties
   d. public panic

10. What is likely to differentiate triage in a public health emergency from triage in a multiple-casualty incident?
    a. types of illness
    b. location of triage sites
    c. viability of patients
    d. availability of personnel

11. Which of the following may be the most ominous deficiency during a public health emergency?
    a. inadequate personnel
    b. scarcity of medical supplies
    c. communications difficulties
    d. public panic

12. Which of the following would most likely cause a delay in response to a public health emergency?
    a. inadequate personnel
    b. scarcity of medical supplies
    c. communications difficulties
    d. public panic

13. Which of the following will help develop critical thinking for managers and supervisory personnel during an emergency?
    a. on-site didactic training
    b. tabletop exercises
    c. on-line MCI exercises
    d. live drills

14. Which of the following can a Paramedic utilize to prepare for a public health emergency while on duty?
    a. on-site didactic training
    b. tabletop exercises
    c. online MCI exercises
    d. live drills

15. Which of the following educational techniques allows both first-line providers and supervisors to interact with systems managers?
    a. on-site didactic training
    b. tabletop exercises
    c. online MCI exercises
    d. live drills

Short Answer

Write a brief answer to each of the following questions.

16. What is the core ethical principle of public health?

_____

_____

17. Describe a public health emergency.

_____

_____

18. What are the challenges to the public health emergency response?

_____

_____

19. What is an "all-hazards" approach?

_____

_____

20. What are some examples of training for a public health emergency?

_____

_____

Fill in the Blank

Complete each sentence by adding the appropriate word in the provided blanks.

21. The first case of an infectious disease is called the _____ _____.

22. A site designated for immunization is called a _____ _____ _____ site.

23. _____ is the physical separation of infected individuals from others.

24. Closing schools, churches, and even movie theaters to prevent the spread of disease is an example of _____ _____.

25. Immunization to prevent the spread of a disease beyond "ground zero" is called _____ _____.

CHAPTER 23

TRIAGE SYSTEMS

Case Study

Smoke continues to bellow from the apartment complex. The buildings have been evacuated and all of the occupants are either in the commandeered city buses or under the awning of the only building not on fire.

"You two!" yells the operations leader. "Take a team and start to set up triage." The two Paramedics look at each other, look at the assembled band of EMS providers from five different services, and look at the operations leader again. "What triage system do you want us to use?" they wonder.

Critical Thinking Questions

1. What is the first type of triage that the Paramedics would use?

   _____

   _____

2. What are the disadvantages of this first triage?

   _____

   _____

"But, sir," the young EMT protests. "I've never done this before and I'm not sure that I am comfortable deciding who lives or dies!" The operations leader replies, "Sure, it's hard, but no triage is triage as well. Just do your best and later you can feel comfortable in your efforts."

"But what if I make a mistake?" asks the EMT. "No worries," replies the operations leader. "You are only the first triage. There will be many more down the line and they will pick out your mistake and correct it. But we have got to get going, NOW!"

Critical Thinking Questions

3. What are some complications of inappropriate triage?

   _____

   _____

4. Name a problem associated with the START triage.

   _____

   _____

Practice Questions

Multiple Choice

Select the best answer for each of the following questions.

1. Which of the following is considered to be the first civilian triage system?
   a. Simple Triage and Rapid Transport (START) system
   b. Sort–Assess–Lifesaving interventions–Treat/transport (SALT) triage system
   c. Sacco Triage and Resource Methodology (STM)
   d. Secondary Assessment of Victim Endpoint (SAVE)

2. What differentiates JumpSTART from START?
   a. ambulatory status
   b. respiratory status
   c. palpable pulses
   d. level of consciousness

3. Which triage system directs the triage officer to reposition the patient's airway?
   a. START system
   b. SALT system
   c. Emergency Severity Index (ESI) system
   d. SAVE system

4. Which triage system does NOT have an expectant category?
   a. START system
   b. SALT system
   c. STM system
   d. SAVE system

5. Which triage system was developed by the Centers for Disease Control and Prevention?
   a. START system
   b. SALT system
   c. STM system
   d. SAVE system

6. Which system is designed on evidence-based research?
   a. START system
   b. SALT system
   c. STM system
   d. SAVE system

7. Which system has two steps?
   a. START system
   b. SALT system
   c. STM system
   d. SAVE system

8. Which system has five steps?
   a. START system
   b. SALT system
   c. STM system
   d. SAVE system

9. Which system uses a total score rather than an algorithmic approach?
   a. START system
   b. SALT system
   c. STM system
   d. SAVE system

10. Which system has been evaluated in an actual disaster?
    a. START system
    b. SALT system
    c. STM system
    d. SAVE system

11. Which system is most effective in a public health emergency?
    a. START system
    b. SALT system
    c. STM system
    d. SAVE system

12. Which system provides treatment priorities instead of transport priorities?
    a. START system
    b. SALT system
    c. STM system
    d. SAVE system

13. Which triage is used in emergency departments?
    a. Canadian Triage and Acuity Scale (CTAS)
    b. SALT system
    c. ESI
    d. SAVE system

14. Which triage system takes into account a diagnosis?
    a. CTAS
    b. SALT system
    c. ESI
    d. SAVE system

15. Which triage system takes pediatrics into account?
    a. CTAS
    b. SALT system
    c. ESI
    d. JumpSTART

Short Answer

Write a brief answer to each of the following questions.

16. What is the goal of triage?

   _____

   _____

17. When did the paradigm shift from the "worst first" to the "greatest good for the greatest number"?

   _____

   _____

18. Describe the SALT system of triage.

_____

_____

19. What triage system uses evidence-based triage methodology?

_____

_____

20. Is triage performed only once?

_____

_____

Fill in the Blank

Complete each sentence by adding the appropriate word in the provided blanks.

21. The first triage scheme, advocated by Baron Larrey, was _____ _____.

22. Underestimating a patient's injuries is an example of _____.

23. Overestimating the criticality of a patient's wounds is an example of _____.

24. Patients with mortal wounds are classified _____.

25. Pediatric triage is done using _____.

CHAPTER 24

VEHICLE RESCUE AND EXTRICATION

Case Study

The tiny hybrid looks like it was rolled over by the pickup truck. Even though the car is destroyed, Buck knows that the occupants might be alive and unharmed inside the shell of the wreckage. "These cars are designed to implode," Buck explains to the new EMT. Seeing his puzzled look, Buck clarifies, "It takes the energy of the crash into the car frame and away from the driver."

Critical Thinking Questions

1. What are the Paramedic's first responsibilities on the scene of a motor vehicle collision?

_____

_____

2. What are the initial actions the Paramedic should take to immobilize the vehicle?

_____

_____

With the door popped, thanks to the rescue boys, and the steering column pushed back, Buck is able to get the backboard under the patient's "hinder-ender," as he calls it. Over his shoulder he can see a couple of new firefighters looking for something under the hood. "Be careful there," instructs Buck. "This is a hybrid. Cut the wrong wire and you could get fried!"

Critical Thinking Questions

3. What are some typical "space-making" techniques that a Paramedic can implement prior to the arrival of heavy rescue?

_____

_____

4. What are the implications of new hybrid drivetrains?

_____

_____

Practice Questions

Multiple Choice

Select the best answer for each of the following questions.

1. Which National Fire Protection Association standard describes the levels of vehicle rescue?
   a. 472
   b. 1670
   c. 1974
   d. 1999

2. Which level of responder is expected to perform extrication?
   a. Awareness
   b. Operations
   c. Technician
   d. Expert

3. Which level of responder is expected to recognize the need for vehicle rescue?
   a. Awareness
   b. Operations
   c. Technician
   d. Expert

4. Which level of responder is expected to perform a risk-benefit analysis?
   a. Awareness
   b. Operations
   c. Technician
   d. Expert

5. Which level is expected to have the same core competencies as needed for hazardous materials?
   a. Awareness
   b. Operations
   c. Technician
   d. Expert

6. Which of the following is NOT part of the Paramedic's efforts to mitigate hazards on the scene of a motor vehicle crash?
   a. Identify the vehicle.
   b. Immobilize the vehicle.
   c. Stabilize the vehicle.
   d. Disable the vehicle.

7. The National Fire Protection Association recommends a _____ circle be established around the vehicle as the "action circle" or the "hot zone."
   a. 6 feet
   b. 12 feet
   c. 15 feet
   d. 20 feet

8. Use of a crowbar to dislodge a door is an example of which process?
   a. disentanglement
   b. space making
   c. extrication
   d. heavy rescue

9. A long-axis drag onto a backboard is an example of which process?
   a. disentanglement
   b. space making
   c. extrication
   d. heavy rescue

10. Flapping the roof to gain access is an example of which process?
    a. disentanglement
    b. space making
    c. extrication
    d. heavy rescue

11. Which of the following is NOT a characteristic of Paramedic extrication gear?
    a. breathable to reduce heat load
    b. offers protection from fluid contamination
    c. resistant to abrasions
    d. fireproof

12. Which of the following is NOT required by the ANSI/ISEA 207 (2006)?
    a. 450 square inches of fluorescent material
    b. 100% color orange or lime-green
    c. 200 square inches of reflective material
    d. 360 degrees of reflectivity

13. Which of the following is an example of hard protection?
    a. placing a short board between the patient and the power cutters
    b. placing a helmet on the patient's head
    c. placing a jam strut to prevent vehicle collapse
    d. placing a sheet of contact paper over the windows

14. Which of the following "space-making" techniques is NOT performed by the Paramedic?
    a. tilting the steering wheel
    b. rolling down the window
    c. sliding the seat back
    d. rolling the dashboard

15. What color is the automotive standard for high-voltage wires?
    a. red
    b. yellow
    c. orange
    d. blue

Short Answer

Write a brief answer to each of the following questions.

16. Differentiate disentanglement from extrication.

_____

_____

17. What is ROPS?

_____

_____

18. Describe a modified dash roll.

_____

_____

19. What is one of the most effective methods of space making?

_____

_____

20. What is a hybrid drivetrain?

_____

_____

Fill in the Blank

Complete each sentence by adding the appropriate word in the provided blanks.

21. Personal protective equipment, including turnout style coats and helmets, is an example of creating a _____ _____ for the Paramedic.

22. The keys for cars with automatic starters should be placed at least _____ feet away from the vehicle.

23. A _____ _____ uses hydrogen and methanol to make electricity.

24. Driver and passenger airbags, side airbag curtains, and even crash bar airbags are all examples of _____ _____ _____.

25. Powered devices that remove slack from the seat belt are called _____.

CHAPTER 25

EMERGENCY INCIDENT REHABILITATION FOR FIREFIGHTERS

Case Study

"Fire command to Medic 24. Establish a rehabilitation sector in the adjacent structure," the radio barks. The three-story apartment building is fully involved and volunteer fire companies from three townships have arrived onscene.

"How many firefighters do we need to prepare for?" asks Aidan. "Well," Mike says, "That's 10 men to a company, and we have five companies. We're looking at 50 people."

Critical Thinking Questions

1. What are the two philosophical components of the rehabilitation standard?

   _____

   _____

2. What organizations are covered under the rehabilitation standard?

   _____

   _____

With the rehabilitation sector set up, Aidan prepares for the incoming firefighters. He has at least 20 minutes before he'll see the first firefighter, as the rest are being seen by EMTs who are monitoring them on scene.

However, Aidan's mind is on prevention. "What can we do to prevent heat exhaustion?" he wonders aloud.

Critical Thinking Questions

3. What actions will provide "relief from climatic conditions"?

   _____

   _____

4. What is the most effective active cooling system?

   _____

   _____

Practice Questions

Multiple Choice

Select the best answer for each of the following questions.

1. Which National Fire Protection Association standard discusses prescreening firefighter applicants to determine their fitness for duty?
   a. 1582
   b. 1583
   c. 1584
   d. 1585

2. Which NFPA standard discusses firefighter rehabilitation?
   a. 1582
   b. 1583
   c. 1584
   d. 1585

3. Which NFPA standard discusses fitness programs for firefighters?
   a. 1582
   b. 1583
   c. 1584
   d. 1585

4. Who ultimately determines whether or not a firefighter should return to service?
   a. Paramedic in charge
   b. incident commander
   c. medical authority
   d. law enforcement officer

5. The rehabilitation standard does NOT refer to which of the following individuals?
   a. firefighters
   b. pastoral care
   c. rescue technicians
   d. hazardous materials specialists

6. Which of the following is NOT a recommended interval for firefighter rehabilitation?
   a. following second 30-minute SCBA cylinder
   b. following second 45-minute SCBA cylinder
   c. following first 60-minute SCBA cylinder
   d. following 40 minutes of intense overhaul

7. Which of the following is NOT part of the rehabilitation standard?
   a. relief from climatic conditions
   b. rest and recovery
   c. transportation
   d. member accountability

8. At a minimum, firefighters should be afforded rest for 10 minutes and seen by EMS if they are not adequately rested in _____.
   a. 15 minutes
   b. 20 minutes
   c. 30 minutes
   d. 1 hour

9. Which of the following is NOT considered a passive cooling technique?
   a. removal of turnout gear
   b. application of ice packs
   c. standing in front of a fan
   d. moving to an air-conditioned cab

10. Which of the following is NOT considered an active cooling technique?
    a. forearm immersion
    b. circulating fans
    c. cold towels
    d. misting tents

11. Water loss and dehydration may be best estimated on scene using _____.
    a. urine-specific gravity
    b. pre- and post-operation weight
    c. saliva osmolarity monitors
    d. blood serum osmolarity

12. Firefighters with a complaint of _____ should be seen by a Paramedic.
    a. chest pain
    b. dizziness
    c. dyspnea
    d. all of the above

13. Firefighters observed to have _____ should be seen by a Paramedic.
    a. changes in gait
    b. slurred speech
    c. changes in behavior
    d. all of the above

14. Firefighters with _____, after 20 minutes of rehabilitation, should be seen by a Paramedic.
    a. tachycardia
    b. elevated temperature
    c. hypertension
    d. all of the above

15. Which of the following nail polish colors will NOT give a false reading on the pulse oximeter?
    a. black
    b. blue
    c. green
    d. red

Short Answer

Write a brief answer to each of the following questions.

16. NFPA 1584 standards in the 2008 version are based on what premise?

   _____

   _____

17. Define rehabilitation.

   _____

   _____

18. Describe the setup for a cold towel cooling system.

_____

_____

19. Define medical monitoring.

_____

_____

20. What is the rehabilitation standard for firefighter accountability?

_____

Fill in the Blank

Complete each sentence by adding the appropriate word in the provided blanks.

21. The _____ _____ should delegate authority to the Paramedic to hold a firefighter in rehabilitation if, in the Paramedic's professional judgment, the firefighter should not be allowed to return to service.

22. The rehabilitation sector officer should utilize atmospheric information and either the _____ _____ index, in the cold, or the _____ _____ index in heat.

23. The ideal fluid for rehydration following dehydration is _____.

24. Emergency scenes lasting more than _____ hours may require the provision of calorie and/or electrolyte replacement.

25. The observation of a firefighter for adverse effects of firefighting is called _____ _____.

CHAPTER 26

HAZARDOUS MATERIALS OPERATIONS

Case Study

Joe's old flower shed is ablaze when the first fire units arrive. While the fire department starts establishing a perimeter, the chief's main concern is the chemical fertilizers and other potentially hazardous materials inside the building.

From his command post, the chief can see the placard on the building. Handing the binoculars to the EMS supervisor, he says, "I see trouble in the form of a vapor cloud."

Critical Thinking Questions

1. What will help the first responder identify the contents of the building?

   _____

   _____

2. Why would knowing the vapor density of the burning material be important?

   _____

   _____

The EMS supervisor has just set up the rehabilitation sector when Incident Command relates that there may be some people down inside the building. "Better gear up the decontamination corridor. I sent a runner over with the MSDS sheet we salvaged from the front office. Better learn everything you can while I look up the IDLH. We need to determine what chance of survival those people have."

Critical Thinking Questions

3. What information does the IDLH (Immediately Dangerous to Life and Health) system provide?

   _____

   _____

4. What are the advantages of on-scene decontamination?

   _____

   _____

Practice Questions

Multiple Choice

Select the best answer for each of the following questions.

1. What level of responder do all responders need to attain?
   a. Awareness level
   b. Operations level
   c. Technician level
   d. Specialist level

2. What level of responder responds to a hazardous materials incident, dons personal protective equipment, and controls the spill?
   a. Awareness level
   b. Operations level
   c. Technician level
   d. Specialist level

3. What level of responder is responsible for implementing the decontamination procedures?
   a. Awareness level
   b. Operations level
   c. Technician level
   d. Specialist level

4. What level of responder is responsible for control of the scene?
   a. Awareness level
   b. Operations level
   c. Technician level
   d. Specialist level

5. Which National Fire Protection Association standard provides for competency of responders?
   a. NFPA 471
   b. NFPA 472
   c. NFPA 473
   d. NFPA 474

6. What National Fire Protection Association standard provides for EMS response?
   a. NFPA 471
   b. NFPA 472
   c. NFPA 473
   d. NFPA 474

7. Which container carrier is oval or elliptical and not under pressure?
   a. MC306
   b. MC307
   c. MC312
   d. MC338

8. Which container carrier carries corrosives under low pressures?
   a. MC306
   b. MC307
   c. MC312
   d. MC338

9. Which container carrier looks like a thermos bottle?
   a. MC306
   b. MC307
   c. MC312
   d. MC338

10. Which container carrier, sometimes called a "bluntie," is double hulled and carries chemicals under low pressure?
    a. MC306
    b. MC307
    c. MC312
    d. MC338

11. Which section of the *Emergency Response Guidebook* contains first aid information?
    a. white section
    b. green section
    c. yellow section
    d. orange section

12. What does the "P" next to the hazardous materials listing on a placard mean?
    a. potentially explosive
    b. potent carcinogen
    c. polymerization
    d. powerful

13. Protective distances (i.e., evacuation) are contained in which section of the *Emergency Response Guidebook*?
    a. white section
    b. green section
    c. yellow section
    d. orange section

14. The white section of the NFPA 704 placard is for what topic?
    a. special hazards
    b. explosive danger
    c. fire warning
    d. flammability

15. What concentration of a chemical will kill 50% of the people exposed to it?
    a. lethal dose
    b. fatal concentration
    c. lethal concentration
    d. threshold limit

Short Answer

Write a brief answer to each of the following questions.

16. Define hazardous materials.

   _____

   _____

17. Define what is meant by a compressed gas.

   _____

   _____

18. What is vapor density?

_____

_____

19. Explain threshold limit values-short-term exposure limit.

_____

_____

20. What are the elements of medical surveillance?

_____

_____

Fill in the Blank

Complete each sentence by adding the appropriate word in the provided blanks.

21. The _____ _____ _____ is a common resource for all emergency responders to hazardous materials incidents.

22. The _____ _____ is the minimum temperature whereby the chemical evaporates at a rate sufficient to ignite.

23. The _____ _____ _____ occurs when the fuel and air mixture is lean (i.e., too much air) and will not support combustion.

24. The _____ _____ _____ occurs when the fuel and air mixture is too rich (i.e., more fuel than air) and will not support combustion.

25. Chemicals that have flammable vapors that self-ignite are called _____.

CHAPTER 27

URBAN SEARCH AND RESCUE

Case Study

The carnage in Haiti made Jose think about joining the USAR team. He had heard about them from John, one of the Paramedics in the department. So, he and John sat down to have a cup of coffee.

"Well, first, our team is not allowed off U.S. soil," John explains. Jose is surprised! "What about Haitian relief?" Jose asks. John explains about the Federal Response Plan, the place of Urban Search and Rescue in that plan, and suggests Jose attend their next meeting to find out more.

Critical Thinking Questions

1. Under what authority does federal Urban Search and Rescue operate?

_____

_____

2. How many USAR teams are there?

_____

_____

After their coffee, Jose goes for a walk to consider what he had heard. He feels he has plenty to offer a USAR. He was an experienced heavy equipment operator before becoming a Paramedic, and USAR will offer him a chance for more training and experience. Plus, the duty cycle works out so as to not put too much strain on the family. He decides to take up John's offer to attend the next USAR meeting to meet some of the folks and to get a closer look at the operation.

Critical Thinking Questions

3. How does the technical USAR team operate?

_____

_____

4. How does the medical USAR team operate?

_____

_____

Practice Questions

Multiple Choice

Select the best answer for each of the following questions.

1. Urban Search and Rescue (USAR) falls under Emergency Support Function 9: _____ of the Federal Response Plan.
   a. Search and Rescue
   b. Medical Support
   c. Operations
   d. Logistic Support

2. Where are the largest numbers of USAR teams found?
   a. California
   b. Surrounding Washington, DC
   c. New York City
   d. Florida

3. What is the only USAR team permitted to deploy outside of the United States?
   a. Los Angeles Task Force One
   b. Pennsylvania Task Force One
   c. Virginia Task Force One
   d. United States Army Task Force

4. How often do USAR teams rotate "first-due" in their district?
   a. every month
   b. every three months
   c. twice annually
   d. annually

5. What is a notice to prepare for a response to a deployment called?
   a. advisory
   b. alert
   c. activation
   d. attention

6. A limited response is seen with a _____ response.
   a. Type I
   b. Type II
   c. Type III
   d. Type IV

7. _____ use specialized computers, microphones, fiber-optic cameras, and so on, for Urban Search and Rescue.
   a. technical search operators
   b. USAR specialists
   c. audio-optical engineers
   d. incident support team members

8. What is a typical canine used for a USAR team?
   a. German shepherd
   b. bloodhound
   c. beagle
   d. labrador retriever

9. Which of the following is NOT part of the technical USAR team?
   a. hazardous materials specialists
   b. structural specialists
   c. heavy equipment specialists
   d. medical specialists

10. Only physicians and _____ are part of the medical USAR team.
    a. Paramedics
    b. nurses
    c. physician assistants
    d. pharmacists

11. Which of the following certifications is NOT needed by Paramedics?
    a. PALS
    b. ACLS
    c. CPR
    d. PHTLS

12. Which of the following conditions is NOT a result of crush syndrome?
    a. rhabdomyolysis
    b. hyperkalemia
    c. renal failure
    d. hypervolemia

13. What usually causes immediate death on scene following a crush injury?
    a. hypovolemia
    b. acidosis
    c. hyperkalemia
    d. hypocalcemia

14. What is the treatment of choice for crush injury?
    a. forced diuresis
    b. alkalinization of the urine
    c. removal of potassium
    d. all of the above

15. The disaster response search and rescue team is capable of being completely self-sustaining for what period of time?
    a. 24 hours
    b. 48 hours
    c. 72 hours
    d. 96 hours

Short Answer

Write a brief answer to each of the following questions.

16. Define confined space.

   _____

   _____

17. Differentiate heavy and light construction.

   _____

   _____

18. Define rostered three deep.

_____

_____

19. Differentiate a rescue from a recovery.

_____

_____

20. What specialists are on a technical team?

_____

_____

Fill in the Blank

Complete each sentence by adding the appropriate word in the provided blanks.

21. A Type _____ response deploys a full team with four canines and all equipment.

22. _____ _____ use diamond chain saws, exothermic torches, and breakers.

23. Physicians serve as _____ _____ _____, and Paramedics are _____
_____.

24. An effort to save a life is called a _____, whereas an effort to retrieve a body is called a _____.

25. Prolonged force to an entrapped limb results in _____ _____.

CHAPTER **28**

WATER RESCUE

Case Study

Heavy spring rains have swollen the river to dangerous levels. Several kayakers, sick of the winter doldrums, are eager to hit the water despite the warnings of local law enforcement. A few hours later, a report of a kayak found floating without a kayaker crosses the sheriff's desk. He sighs, as this seems to happen every spring—at least, it had for as long as he could remember,

Critical Thinking Questions

1. What are the types of water rescue?

   _____

   _____

2. What are the different types of water search methods?

   _____

   _____

The sheriff's deputies are familiar with the drill. First, they contact the sheriff's departments in the neighboring towns. The sheriff's department in the next county, being larger and having access to more resources, offers a swift water rescue team complete with fast water boats.

   Next, the deputies interview witnesses, establish the patient's point last seen (PLS), and start establishing Incident Command for the inevitable search. However, they know that, in some unfortunate instances, these rescues turn into a recovery operation instead.

Critical Thinking Questions

3. What are the dangers in swift water rescue?

   _____

   _____

4. What safety measures are taken during a swift water rescue?

   _____

   _____

Practice Questions

Multiple Choice

Select the best answer for each of the following questions.

1. What is water moving at less than one knot called?
   a. calm water
   b. swift water
   c. flat water
   d. surface water

2. A hydraulic current creates a "killing machine." Where are hydraulic currents found?
   a. low-head dams
   b. flood control reservoir outlets
   c. storm drains
   d. earthen dams

3. What is the strongest ice?
   a. clear ice
   b. river ice
   c. consolidated ice
   d. rotten ice

4. What are the most dangerous waves?
   a. spilling waves
   b. surging waves
   c. plunging waves
   d. tumbling waves

5. Which water flows push water perpendicular to the shore?
   a. rip currents
   b. surging waves
   c. hydraulic currents
   d. spilling waves

6. Which NFPA standard pertains to team operations and training?
   a. NFPA 1006
   b. NFPA 1670
   c. NFPA 1999
   d. NFPA 1010

7. Which level of training is needed, minimally, to use shore-based rescue?
   a. Level II
   b. Operations level
   c. Level I
   d. Technical rescuers

8. What classification of personal flotation device is most commonly used by fire, EMS, and law enforcement rescue?
   a. Type 1
   b. Type 2
   c. Type 3
   d. Type 4

9. What classification of personal flotation device is generally used by a swift water rescuer?
   a. Type 2
   b. Type 3
   c. Type 4
   d. Type 5

10. What other equipment, besides a personal flotation device, is the minimum needed for swift water rescue?
    a. helmets
    b. whistles
    c. water knives
    d. personal throw bags

11. Lying facedown in the water, without moving the hands and legs, and only lifting the head to breathe describes which of the following positions?
    a. drownproofing position
    b. self-rescue position
    c. heat escape lessening position
    d. defensive swimming position

12. What is water piling up on a submerged object called?
    a. upstream V
    b. strainer
    c. pillow
    d. downstream V

13. When the rescuer is caught in a rip current, how should the rescuer swim in relation to the current?
    a. against the current
    b. out away from the current
    c. under the current
    d. perpendicular to the current

14. Which of the following situations is NOT likely to prompt a passive search?
    a. failure to report back in time with a boat
    b. boat found abandoned in a lake
    c. swimmer overboard
    d. boat wreckage

15. Which of the following is NOT a tool used in shore-based rescue?
    a. Sheppard's crook
    b. throw bag
    c. ring buoy
    d. boat gunnels

Short Answer

Write a brief answer to each of the following questions.

16. What is differential pressure?

_____

_____

17. What is the defensive swimming position to use when one is suddenly caught in fast water?

_____

_____

18. What is the greatest danger to rescuers in fast water?

_____

_____

19. What is the greatest danger to rescuers in surf rescue?

_____

_____

20. What is triangulation?

_____

_____

Fill in the Blank

Complete each sentence by adding the appropriate word in the provided blanks.

21. The most dangerous dam is a _____ _____ dam because of its _____ _____.

22. The most dangerous waves in the surf are _____ _____.

23. Whenever a rescuer is near the water, the rescuer should have a _____ _____ _____.

24. When immersed in water that is colder than body temperature, the rescuer should assume the _____ _____ _____ _____.

25. Downed trees and branches create _____ in a river or stream.

CHAPTER 29

WILDERNESS SEARCH AND RESCUE

Case Study

The North Franklin volunteer fire department is called out to find two individuals "lost" in the Black Hills area. The firefighters have recently completed their search and rescue courses, provided by the local forest ranger. Under the command of the state police, they are now being sent to a staging area.

While bouncing down the bumpy dirt road, Jon, an experienced search and rescue technician, is adjusting his gear and listening to the chatter of the radio.

Critical Thinking Questions

1. What National Fire Protection Association standard relates to wilderness search and rescue?

   _____

   _____

2. What are the levels of SAR responders?

   _____

   _____

Fortunately, the couple has left plenty of clues, and Jon can establish a general direction of travel based on the point last seen. If they followed the pattern of many lost persons, Jon assumes the couple started to follow the streams, hoping to find a bridge or a road. Unfortunately, the couple would not know that cliffs lie ahead. "One slip is all it takes," Jon says to the assembled responders. "Theirs or ours. Let's be mindful of the footing as well as conscious of the clues."

With those words of wisdom, the first three-person team heads down the trail to perform a hasty search. In the interim, a team with a pointer and some flankers are standing by, waiting for the first word of a fresh clue.

Critical Thinking Questions

3. What are the rudimentary searches performed at the beginning of the search and rescue operation?

   _____

   _____

4. What is tracking?

   _____

   _____

Practice Questions

Multiple Choice

Select the best answer for each of the following questions.

1. Which of the following is NOT a goal for search and rescue operations?
   a. locate
   b. stabilize with medical care
   c. debrief
   d. transport to definitive care

2. The Paramedic at the _____ level is expected to recognize the need for wilderness search and rescue.
   a. Awareness
   b. Operations
   c. Technician
   d. Specialist

3. The Paramedic at the _____ level is trained in rope rescue.
   a. Awareness
   b. Operations
   c. Technician
   d. Specialist

4. Land navigation includes use of which of the following tools?
   a. map and compass
   b. geographical information system
   c. global positioning satellites
   d. all of the above

5. Which of the following is NOT an indirect search tactic?
   a. attraction
   b. containment
   c. hasty search
   d. fact finding

6. Which of the following is NOT a direct search tactic?
   a. aerial reconnaissance
   b. loose grid searches
   c. canine searches
   d. global positioning satellite

7. Who usually performs hasty searches?
   a. Type I searchers
   b. Awareness level searchers
   c. first responders
   d. triage

8. All of the following searches are intended to yield clues, not necessarily find the patient, EXCEPT _____.
   a. tight grid search
   b. hasty search
   c. loose grid search
   d. bastard search

9. Which of the following would NOT be considered a direct clue?
   a. footprints
   b. summit flags
   c. witness testimony
   d. smoke

10. Which of the following is NOT used by the sign cutter?
    a. cutting stick
    b. compass
    c. bracketing
    d. pointer

11. Which of the following is NOT an example of a natural sign?
    a. disturbed soil
    b. articles of clothing
    c. scratches on rock
    d. path in the dew

12. Who are the most unpredictable patients?
    a. children 1 to 3 years
    b. children 3 to 6 years
    c. children 6 to 12 years
    d. children 12 to 18 years

13. Which patients are likely to run away?
    a. children 1 to 3 years
    b. children 3 to 6 years
    c. children 6 to 12 years
    d. children 12 to 18 years

14. Which patients are likely to get lost "on purpose"?
    a. elderly
    b. mentally challenged
    c. autistic
    d. despondent

15. Which patients are likely to be found in an idyllic spot?
    a. elderly
    b. mentally challenged
    c. autistic
    d. despondent

Short Answer

Write a brief answer to each of the following questions.

16. Statistically, what is the greatest predictor of survival for a lost person?

_____

_____

17. What is a hasty search?

_____

_____

18. What is a bastard search?

_____

_____

19. What is clue consciousness?

_____

_____

20. What is sign cutting?

_____

_____

Fill in the Blank

Complete each sentence by adding the appropriate word in the provided blanks.

21. The area where the patient will most likely be found is called the _____ _____
    _____.

22. The start of every search occurs at the _____ _____ _____.

23. A cut in the boot of a searcher is called the _____ _____.

24. The sudden onset of overwhelming panic at the realization of being lost is called _____
    _____.

25. A new and necessary part of the EMS role in wilderness search and rescue operations is _____
    _____.

CHAPTER 30

TECHNICAL ROPE RESCUE

Case Study

"Janet and Laura!" Chief Erb calls out. "I want you two to start the information gathering phase of our technical rescue team. We have an opportunity to secure a grant and I need the basic information to make our case. You can start with a hazard analysis."

"I don't need to remind you that money is tight," Chief Erb continues. "So use your wits and use your resources to complete the task, but do it cheaply. If you have any questions, ask Dennis. He's the man with the know-how to do this."

Critical Thinking Questions

1. What is a hazard analysis?

   _____

   _____

2. What is a slope analysis?

   _____

   _____

Janet turns to Laura and asks, "Where do we go first?"

"Well," Laura replies. "Let's look at the National Fire Protection Association standards. We are not the first to do this and I will bet that the standards will help guide us." "Yes," Janet agrees. "We need to think comprehensively, considering things like training equipment—everything right down to the ropes!"

Critical Thinking Questions

3. What National Fire Protection Association standards relate to operations and training for technical rescue?

   _____

   _____

4. What National Fire Protection Association standards relate to technical rescue equipment?

   _____

   _____

Practice Questions
Multiple Choice

1. Which of the following is included in the hazard analysis?
   a. water tower
   b. multistory building
   c. farm silo
   d. all of the above

2. When the rescuer's weight is on her feet, it is called a _____ angle rescue.
   a. slope
   b. low
   c. steep
   d. highline

3. When the rescuer's entire weight is on the rope, it is called a _____ angle rescue.
   a. slope
   b. low
   c. steep
   d. highline

4. Which National Fire Protection Association standard specifically deals with rescue operations?
   a. NFPA 1006
   b. NFPA 1670
   c. NFPA 1983
   d. NFPA 1999

5. Which National Fire Protection Association standard specifically deals with ropes and rope safety?
   a. NFPA 1006
   b. NFPA 1670
   c. NFPA 1983
   d. NFPA 1999

6. Which National Fire Protection Association standard specifically deals with levels of rescue training?
   a. NFPA 1006
   b. NFPA 1670
   c. NFPA 1983
   d. NFPA 1999

7. A full body harness (i.e., shoulders and pelvis) is a _____ harness.
   a. Class I
   b. Class II
   c. Class III
   d. Class IV

8. A self-rescue harness is a _____ harness.
   a. Class I
   b. Class II
   c. Class III
   d. Class IV

9. Which of the following ropes is NOT used for rescue?
   a. dynamic rope
   b. low stretch rope
   c. true static rope
   d. kernmantle

10. Which of the following carabiners is NOT used in rescue?
    a. D-shaped
    b. locking
    c. steel
    d. single oval

11. Which of the following descent devices is typically used only during an emergency?
    a. figure eight
    b. reverse ascender
    c. brake bar
    d. prusik knot

12. To "tie in," the _____ knot is used.
    a. figure eight
    b. granny
    c. square
    d. woodsman's bend

13. Which command means, "Are you ready?"
    a. on rappel
    b. rappel on?
    c. tension
    d. rope free

14. Which of the following materials is NOT used to make rescue baskets?
    a. fiberglass
    b. wire mesh
    c. Kevlar
    d. canvas

15. Rescuers each taking a corner of the rescue basket is called the _____ carry.
    a. four-corner
    b. diamond
    c. overland
    d. caterpillar

Short Answer

Write a brief answer to each of the following questions.

16. What ropes are designated for rescue?

_____

_____

17. What is a belay?

_____

_____

18. What is mechanical advantage?

_____

_____

19. What is the most effective hauling system?

_____

_____

20. What prevents the patient from falling out of the basket?

_____

_____

Fill in the Blank

Complete each sentence by adding the appropriate word on the provided blanks.

21. Rescue over a chasm or ravine is called _____.

22. A _____ _____ permits multiple carabiners to be attached.

23. Descent (i.e., rappelling) is controlled with a _____ _____ _____.

24. The _____ _____ _____ spreads the patient's weight over several points.

25. A loop of webbing attached to the basket that helps with lifting is called a _____.

CHAPTER 31

MASS-GATHERING MEDICINE

Case Study

"Duke," says the chief. "The stamp collectors' bazaar is coming up! Remember last year? We had over two dozen elderly patients overcome by the heat! Let's not have a repeat of that this year. I have decided to task you with preplanning this year's events at the county fairgrounds and I want a plan within a week."

Critical Thinking Questions

1. What aspects should be considered in event preplanning?

   _____

   _____

2. What is the role of public health?

   _____

   _____

"Chief," Duke asks, "what kind of resources do I have? Do I have extra personnel or do I have to make due with the on-duty personnel? Can I call in the area volunteers, like the Medical Reserve Corps? And what about supplies and equipment? Do we have any equipment caches?"

"Well, son," the chief explains. "It seems like you've got a lot of homework to do!"

Critical Thinking Questions

3. What are examples of "early warning systems" for medical emergencies?

   _____

   _____

4. What on-scene care should be available?

   _____

   _____

Practice Questions
Multiple Choice

Select the best answer for each of the following questions.

1. Which of the following should be taken into account when planning for a mass-gathering event?
   a. biomedical factors
   b. psychosocial factors
   c. environmental factors
   d. all of the above

2. Which of the following is NOT an environmental factor?
   a. location
   b. indoors versus outdoors
   c. weather forecast
   d. anticipated crowds

3. At which of the following events is the patient load anticipated to be highest?
   a. rock concert
   b. marathon
   c. old song festival
   d. sporting event

4. Which of the following actions at a rock concert can cause head trauma?
   a. mosh pits
   b. body surfing
   c. slam dancing
   d. all of the above

5. Which of the following people help to decrease the litigation profile?
   a. event planners
   b. risk managers
   c. venue managers
   d. law enforcement

6. Which of the following are used to prevent heat exhaustion at a mass gathering?
   a. pallets of water
   b. fog streams over the crowd
   c. tents for shade
   d. all of the above

7. Which of the following is NOT a role of public health?
   a. medical care
   b. food safety
   c. water inspection
   d. waste management

8. Which of the following personnel does NOT need to be at the Emergency Operations Center?
   a. incident commander
   b. public information officer
   c. safety officer
   d. operations officer

9. Which of the following is NOT a common complaint at a mass gathering?
   a. headache
   b. blisters
   c. chest pain
   d. sunburn

10. Which of the following can offer assistance at mass gatherings?
    a. Disaster Assistance Response Teams
    b. Disaster Medical Assistance Teams
    c. Medical Reserve Corps.
    d. all of the above

11. To improve the patient's survival in cardiac arrest, it is important to have which of the following?
    a. CPR-trained first responders
    b. seamless communications chain
    c. strategically placed AED
    d. all of the above

12. Which of the following is NOT part of an event profile?
    a. type of event
    b. restricted versus extended
    c. crowd sentiment
    d. on-site transportation

13. Which of the following is NOT a device used for on-site transportation?
    a. four-wheeled carts
    b. modified golf carts
    c. ambulances
    d. wheelchairs

14. Which of the following is NOT part of human surveillance?
    a. untrained civilian spotters
    b. roving teams
    c. cameras
    d. forward aid station

15. Which of the following is considered a form of "surge" protection for the hospitals?
    a. forward aid station
    b. triage
    c. ambulance stacking
    d. field hospital

Short Answer

Write a brief answer to each of the following questions.

16. What is the goal of mass-gathering medicine?

_____

_____

17. Describe the techniques for effective alcohol management (TEAM).

_____

_____

18. Describe the human stampede.

_____

_____

19. What are the steps for mass evacuation following a credible threat of weapons of mass destruction?

_____

_____

20. What is an event profile?

_____

_____

Fill in the Blank

Complete each sentence by adding the appropriate word in the provided blanks.

21. The National Association of EMS Physicians and American College of Emergency Physicians say a group of more than _____ constitutes a mass gathering.

22. The emotional tone set by an event directly relates to the _____ _____.

23. Medical emergencies per 1,000 attendees is called the _____ _____.

24. Crowd crush is also known as _____ _____.

25. With the danger of weapons of mass destruction, event planners must consider _____ _____.

CHAPTER 32

TACTICAL EMERGENCY MEDICAL SUPPORT

Case Study

"Doc, the police department has asked the fire department to assign one of its firefighter–medics to the tactical operations team," says the fire chief. "Naturally, with your military background as a medic and soldier you seem like a natural fit. However, we don't have the resources to reassign you to the police permanently. Therefore, you are on temporary assignment. Understand?"

Nick considers the request for a moment. He understands the mission, he is capable of performing the mission, and he knows that eventually he may be able to work it into a permanent assignment. "Yes, sir," Nick replies. "Assignment accepted."

Critical Thinking Questions

1. What are the four missions of the tactical medic?

   _____

   _____

2. What are the advantages of hospital-based medical support? EMS/Fire-based medical support? Law enforcement-based medical support?

   _____

   _____

"Welcome, Doc, to the other side of the house," quips the police chief. "You will be called up for special duty whenever the SWAT goes out. Warrant service, snipers, hostages, you know, that kind of stuff. But I want you to keep your head down. The fire chief told me if I lose you then I have to send him two cops to replace you," the chief chuckles at his joke. "What do you need to get started?"

Critical Thinking Questions

3. If EMS is not medically trained, then under what conditions must its members operate at the scene of a tactical operation?

   _____

   _____

4. What is the minimum equipment needed for a Paramedic to operate in the cool zone?

   _____

   _____

Practice Questions

Multiple Choice

Select the best answer for each of the following questions.

1. Which of the following is NOT an example of a current tactical EMS unit?
   a. law-enforcement based
   b. military based
   c. Fire/EMS based
   d. hospital based

2. Who does the majority of medical support for tactical law enforcement operations?
   a. civilian EMS
   b. military EMS
   c. law enforcement EMS
   d. none of the above

3. Which of the following is NOT part of the special body of knowledge that a tactical medic must possess?
   a. weapons safety
   b. hazardous materials
   c. psychological counseling
   d. advanced physiology

4. Which of the following is NOT part of the medical threat assessment?
   a. determination of mission objective
   b. potential environmental exposure
   c. determination of safe landing zones
   d. weather forecast

5. Which of the following is NOT special equipment specific to the tactical medic?
   a. cargo pants
   b. ballistic helmet
   c. fireproof balaclava
   d. shatterproof eye protection

6. Which of the following is NOT part of typical self-care for the Paramedic?
   a. gloves
   b. tourniquet
   c. pneumothorax kit
   d. trauma dressing

7. An entry leg bag contains all of the elements of a self-care kit. In addition, it also contains a _____.
   a. pneumothorax kit
   b. cricothyroidotomy kit
   c. intubation kit
   d. minor wound kit

8. In which zone is tactical field care usually provided?
   a. cold zone
   b. cool zone
   c. warm zone
   d. hot zone

9. Medical care in the hot zone primarily consists of which actions?
   a. scoop and run
   b. stay and play
   c. protect in place
   d. suppression and evacuation

10. What usually causes mortality during a tactical operation?
    a. loss of airway
    b. apnea
    c. hemorrhage
    d. internal bleeding

11. Which of the following is NOT a situation that may create a sustained medical operation?
    a. warrant service
    b. hostage scenarios
    c. weapons of mass destruction
    d. sniper attack

12. What term describes providing instructions to others without seeing them?
    a. protect in place
    b. remote medical care
    c. care over the barricade
    d. hostage negotiation

13. What is the lead argument to provide arms to tactical medics?
    a. protect themselves
    b. provide coverage under fire
    c. provide suppressive fire
    d. participate in law enforcement

14. What is the single greatest cause of death on the scene of a tactical operation?
    a. motor vehicle crashes
    b. explosions
    c. gunshot wounds
    d. knife wounds

15. Which of the following is NOT part of the occupational health aspect of tactical medicine?
    a. simple sunburns
    b. ankle sprains
    c. glucose control
    d. gunshot wound

Short Answer

Write a brief answer to each of the following questions.

16. What is tactical EMS?

_____

_____

17. What are the categories of sustained medical operations?

_____

_____

18. What is "care over the barricade"?

_____

_____

19. Differentiate cover from concealment.

_____

_____

20. Describe the concept of "protect in place."

_____

_____

Fill in the Blank

Complete each sentence by adding the appropriate word in the provided blanks.

21. Paramedics trained specifically for the tactical environment are called _____ _____.

22. Reviewing the operation for injury potential is part of the _____ _____ _____.

23. Remaining under cover and providing medical care is called _____ _____ _____.

24. Tactical medics in the warm zone are afforded either _____ _____ or _____ _____ or cover in the warm zone.

25. In the warm zone, the concept of primary assessment is turned on its head and is called the _____ _____ _____.

SECTION II

NREMT SKILLS FOR PARAMEDIC CERTIFICATION

1. Patient Assessment—Medical

2. Patient Assessment—Trauma

3. Ventilatory Management
   - Adult
   - Dual Lumen Airway Device (Combitube® or PTL®)

4. Cardiac Management Skills
   - Dynamic Cardiology
   - Static Cardiology

5. IV and Medication Skills
   - Intravenous Therapy
   - Intravenous Bolus Medications

6. Oral Station

7. Pediatric Skills
   - Pediatric (<2 yrs.) Ventilatory Management
   - Pediatric Intraosseous Infusion

8. Random Basic Skills
   - Spinal Immobilization (Seated Patient)
   - Spinal Immobilization (Supine Patient)
   - Bleeding Control/Shock Management

National Registry of Emergency Medical Technicians
Advanced Level Practical Examination

PATIENT ASSESSMENT - MEDICAL

Candidate: _____ Examiner: _____

Date: _____ Signature: _____

Scenario:_____

	Possible Points	Points Awarded
Time Start: _____		
Takes or verbalizes body substance isolation precautions	1	
SCENE SIZE-UP		
Determines the scene/situation is safe	1	
Determines the mechanism of injury/nature of illness	1	
Determines the number of patients	1	
Requests additional help if necessary	1	
Considers stabilization of spine	1	
INITIAL ASSESSMENT		
Verbalizes general impression of the patient	1	
Determines responsiveness/level of consciousness	1	
Determines chief complaint/apparent life-threats	1	
Assesses airway and breathing 　　-Assessment (1 point) 　　-Assures adequate ventilation (1 point) 　　-Initiates appropriate oxygen therapy (1 point)	3	
Assesses circulation 　　-Assesses/controls major bleeding (1 point)　-Assesses skin [either skin color, temperature, or condition] (1 point) 　　-Assesses pulse (1 point)	3	
Identifies priority patients/makes transport decision	1	
FOCUSED HISTORY AND PHYSICAL EXAMINATION/RAPID ASSESSMENT		
History of present illness 　　-Onset (1 point)　　　　-Severity (1 point) 　　-Provocation (1 point)　　-Time (1 point) 　　-Quality (1 point)　　　-Clarifying questions of associated signs and symptoms as related to OPQRST (2 points) 　　-Radiation (1 point)	8	
Past medical history 　　-Allergies (1 point)　　-Past pertinent history (1 point)　　-Events leading to present illness (1 point) 　　-Medications (1 point)　-Last oral intake (1 point)	5	
Performs focused physical examination [assess affected body part/system or, if indicated, completes rapid assessment] 　　-Cardiovascular　　-Neurological　　　-Integumentary　　-Reproductive 　　-Pulmonary　　　-Musculoskeletal　　-GI/GU　　　　-Psychological/Social	5	
Vital signs 　　-Pulse (1 point)　　　　-Respiratory rate and quality (1 point each) 　　-Blood pressure (1 point)　-AVPU (1 point)	5	
Diagnostics [must include application of ECG monitor for dyspnea and chest pain]	2	
States field impression of patient	1	
Verbalizes treatment plan for patient and calls for appropriate intervention(s)	1	
Transport decision re-evaluated	1	
ON-GOING ASSESSMENT		
Repeats initial assessment	1	
Repeats vital signs	1	
Evaluates response to treatments	1	
Repeats focused assessment regarding patient complaint or injuries	1	
Time End: _____		
CRITICAL CRITERIA　　　　　　　　　　　　　　　**TOTAL**	48	

CRITICAL CRITERIA

_____ Failure to initiate or call for transport of the patient within 15 minute time limit

_____ Failure to take or verbalize body substance isolation precautions

_____ Failure to determine scene safety before approaching patient

_____ Failure to voice and ultimately provide appropriate oxygen therapy

_____ Failure to assess/provide adequate ventilation

_____ Failure to find or appropriately manage problems associated with airway, breathing, hemorrhage or shock [hypoperfusion]

_____ Failure to differentiate patient's need for immediate transportation versus continued assessment and treatment at the scene

_____ Does other detailed or focused history or physical examination before assessing and treating threats to airway, breathing, and circulation

_____ Failure to determine the patient's primary problem

_____ Orders a dangerous or inappropriate intervention

_____ Failure to provide for spinal protection when indicated

You must factually document your rationale for checking any of the above critical items on the reverse side of this form.

Candidate: _____   Examiner: _____

Date: _____   Signature: _____

Scenario # _____

Time Start: _____   NOTE: Areas denoted by "**" may be integrated within sequence of Initial Assessment

	Possible Points	Points Awarded
Takes or verbalizes body substance isolation precautions	1	
SCENE SIZE-UP		
Determines the scene/situation is safe	1	
Determines the mechanism of injury/nature of illness	1	
Determines the number of patients	1	
Requests additional help if necessary	1	
Considers stabilization of spine	1	
INITIAL ASSESSMENT/RESUSCITATION		
Verbalizes general impression of the patient	1	
Determines responsiveness/level of consciousness	1	
Determines chief complaint/apparent life-threats	1	
Airway -Opens and assesses airway (1 point) -Inserts adjunct as indicated (1 point)	2	

Breathing
  -Assess breathing (1 point)
  -Assures adequate ventilation (1 point)
  -Initiates appropriate oxygen therapy (1 point)
  -Manages any injury which may compromise breathing/ventilation (1 point)
	4	

Circulation
  -Checks pulse (1point)
  -Assess skin [either skin color, temperature, or condition] (1 point)
  -Assesses for and controls major bleeding if present (1 point)
  -Initiates shock management (1 point)
	4	

Identifies priority patients/makes transport decision	1	
FOCUSED HISTORY AND PHYSICAL EXAMINATION/RAPID TRAUMA ASSESSMENT		
Selects appropriate assessment	1	
Obtains, or directs assistant to obtain, baseline vital signs	1	
Obtains SAMPLE history	1	
DETAILED PHYSICAL EXAMINATION		

Head
  -Inspects mouth**, nose**, and assesses facial area (1 point)
  -Inspects and palpates scalp and ears (1 point)
  -Assesses eyes for PERRL** (1 point)
	3	

Neck**
  -Checks position of trachea (1 point)
  -Checks jugular veins (1 point)
  -Palpates cervical spine (1 point)
	3	

Chest**
  -Inspects chest (1 point)
  -Palpates chest (1 point)
  -Auscultates chest (1 point)
	3	

Abdomen/pelvis**
  -Inspects and palpates abdomen (1 point)
  -Assesses pelvis (1 point)
  -Verbalizes assessment of genitalia/perineum as needed (1 point)
	3	

Lower extremities** -Inspects, palpates, and assesses motor, sensory, and distal circulatory functions (1 point/leg)	2	
Upper extremities -Inspects, palpates, and assesses motor, sensory, and distal circulatory functions (1 point/arm)	2	

Posterior thorax, lumbar, and buttocks**
  -Inspects and palpates posterior thorax (1 point)
  -Inspects and palpates lumbar and buttocks area (1 point)
	2	

Manages secondary injuries and wounds appropriately	1	
Performs ongoing assessment	1	
TOTAL	**43**	

Time End: _____

CRITICAL CRITERIA

____ Failure to initiate or call for transport of the patient within 10 minute time limit
____ Failure to take or verbalize body substance isolation precautions
____ Failure to determine scene safety
____ Failure to assess for and provide spinal protection when indicated
____ Failure to voice and ultimately provide high concentration of oxygen
____ Failure to assess/provide adequate ventilation
____ Failure to find or appropriately manage problems associated with airway, breathing, hemorrhage or shock [hypoperfusion]
____ Failure to differentiate patient's need for immediate transportation versus continued assessment/treatment at the scene
____ Does other detailed/focused history or physical exam before assessing/treating threats to airway, breathing, and circulation
____ Orders a dangerous or inappropriate intervention

You must factually document your rationale for checking any of the above critical items on the reverse side of this form.

p301/8-003k

VENTILATORY MANAGEMENT - ADULT

Candidate:_____ Examiner:_____

Date: _____ Signature: _____

NOTE: If candidate elects to ventilate initially with BVM attached to reservoir and oxygen, full credit must be awarded for steps denoted by "**" so long as first ventilation is delivered within 30 seconds.

	Possible Points	Points Awarded
Takes or verbalizes body substance isolation precautions	1	
Opens the airway manually	1	
Elevates tongue, inserts simple adjunct [oropharyngeal or nasopharyngeal airway]	1	
NOTE: Examiner now informs candidate no gag reflex is present and patient accepts adjunct		
**Ventilates patient immediately with bag-valve-mask device unattached to oxygen	1	
**Ventilates patient with room air	1	
NOTE: Examiner now informs candidate that ventilation is being performed without difficulty and that pulse oximetry indicates the patient's blood oxygen saturation is 85%		
Attaches oxygen reservoir to bag-valve-mask device and connects to high flow oxygen regulator [12-15 L/minute]	1	
Ventilates patient at a rate of 10-12/minute with appropriate volumes	1	
NOTE: After 30 seconds, examiner auscultates and reports breath sounds are present, equal bilaterally and medical direction has ordered intubation. The examiner must now take over ventilation.		
Directs assistant to pre-oxygenate patient	1	
Identifies/selects proper equipment for intubation	1	
Checks equipment for: -Cuff leaks (1 point) -Laryngoscope operational with bulb tight (1 point)	2	
NOTE: Examiner to remove OPA and move out of the way when candidate is prepared to intubate		
Positions head properly	1	
Inserts blade while displacing tongue	1	
Elevates mandible with laryngoscope	1	
Introduces ET tube and advances to proper depth	1	
Inflates cuff to proper pressure and disconnects syringe	1	
Directs ventilation of patient	1	
Confirms proper placement by auscultation bilaterally over each lung and over epigastrium	1	
NOTE: Examiner to ask, "If you had proper placement, what should you expect to hear?"		
Secures ET tube [may be verbalized]	1	
NOTE: Examiner now asks candidate, "Please demonstrate one additional method of verifying proper tube placement in this patient."		
Identifies/selects proper equipment	1	
Verbalizes findings and interpretations [compares indicator color to the colorimetric scale or EDD recoil and states findings]	1	
NOTE: Examiner now states, "You see secretions in the tube and hear gurgling sounds with the patient's exhalation."		
Identifies/selects a flexible suction catheter	1	
Pre-oxygenates patient	1	
Marks maximum insertion length with thumb and forefinger	1	
Inserts catheter into the ET tube leaving catheter port open	1	
At proper insertion depth, covers catheter port and applies suction while withdrawing catheter	1	
Ventilates/directs ventilation of patient as catheter is flushed with sterile water	1	
TOTAL	**27**	

CRITICAL CRITERIA

_____ Failure to initiate ventilations within 30 seconds after applying gloves or interrupts ventilations for greater than 30 seconds at any time
_____ Failure to take or verbalize body substance isolation precautions
_____ Failure to voice and ultimately provide high oxygen concentrations [at least 85%]
_____ Failure to ventilate patient at a rate of 10 - 12 / minute
_____ Failure to provide adequate volumes per breath [maximum 2 errors/minute permissible]
_____ Failure to pre-oxygenate patient prior to intubation and suctioning
_____ Failure to successfully intubate within 3 attempts
_____ Failure to disconnect syringe **immediately** after inflating cuff of ET tube
_____ Uses teeth as a fulcrum
_____ Failure to assure proper tube placement by auscultation bilaterally **and** over the epigastrium
_____ If used, stylette extends beyond end of ET tube
_____ Inserts any adjunct in a manner dangerous to the patient
_____ Suctions the patient for more than 10 seconds
_____ Does not suction the patient

You must factually document your rationale for checking any of the above critical items on the reverse side of this form.

National Registry of Emergency Medical Technicians
Advanced Level Practical Examination

DUAL LUMEN AIRWAY DEVICE (COMBITUBE® OR PTL®)

Candidate: _____   Examiner: _____

Date: _____   Signature: _____

NOTE: If candidate elects to initially ventilate with BVM attached to reservoir and oxygen, full credit must be awarded for steps denoted by "**" so long as first ventilation is delivered within 30 seconds.

	Possible Points	Points Awarded
Takes or verbalizes body substance isolation precautions	1	
Opens the airway manually	1	
Elevates tongue, inserts simple adjunct [oropharyngeal or nasopharyngeal airway]	1	
NOTE: Examiner now informs candidate no gag reflex is present and patient accepts adjunct		
**Ventilates patient immediately with bag-valve-mask device unattached to oxygen	1	
**Hyperventilates patient with room air	1	
NOTE: Examiner now informs candidate that ventilation is being performed without difficulty		
Attaches oxygen reservoir to bag-valve-mask device and connects to high flow oxygen regulator [12-15 L/minute]	1	
Ventilates patient at a rate of 10-12/minute with appropriate volumes	1	
NOTE: After 30 seconds, examiner auscultates and reports breath sounds are present and equal bilaterally and medical control has ordered insertion of a dual lumen airway. The examiner must now take over ventilation.		
Directs assistant to pre-oxygenate patient	1	
Checks/prepares airway device	1	
Lubricates distal tip of the device [may be verbalized]	1	
NOTE: Examiner to remove OPA and move out of the way when candidate is prepared to insert device		
Positions head properly	1	
Performs a tongue-jaw lift	1	

☐ **USES COMBITUBE®**	☐ **USES PTL®**		
Inserts device in mid-line and to depth so printed ring is at level of teeth	Inserts device in mid-line until bite block flange is at level of teeth	1	
Inflates pharyngeal cuff with proper volume and removes syringe	Secures strap	1	
Inflates distal cuff with proper volume and removes syringe	Blows into tube #1 to adequately inflate both cuffs	1	
Attaches/directs attachment of BVM to the first [esophageal placement] lumen and ventilates		1	
Confirms placement and ventilation through correct lumen by observing chest rise, auscultation over the epigastrium, and bilaterally over each lung		1	

	Possible Points	Points Awarded
NOTE: The examiner states, "You do not see rise and fall of the chest and you only hear sounds over the epigastrium."		
Attaches/directs attachment of BVM to the second [endotracheal placement] lumen and ventilates	1	
Confirms placement and ventilation through correct lumen by observing chest rise, auscultation over the epigastrium, and bilaterally over each lung	1	
NOTE: The examiner confirms adequate chest rise, absent sounds over the epigastrium, and equal bilateral breath sounds.		
Secures device or confirms that the device remains properly secured	1	
TOTAL	**20**	

CRITICAL CRITERIA

_____ Failure to initiate ventilations within 30 seconds after taking body substance isolation precautions or interrupts ventilations for greater than 30 seconds at any time

_____ Failure to take or verbalize body substance isolation precautions

_____ Failure to voice and ultimately provide high oxygen concentrations [at least 85%]

_____ Failure to ventilate patient at a rate of 10-12/minute

_____ Failure to provide adequate volumes per breath [maximum 2 errors/minute permissible]

_____ Failure to pre-oxygenate patient prior to insertion of the dual lumen airway device

_____ Failure to insert the dual lumen airway device at a proper depth or at either proper place within 3 attempts

_____ Failure to inflate both cuffs properly

_____ **Combitube** - failure to remove the syringe immediately after inflation of each cuff

PTL - failure to secure the strap prior to cuff inflation

_____ Failure to confirm that the proper lumen of the device is being ventilated by observing chest rise, auscultation over the epigastrium, and bilaterally over each lung

_____ Inserts any adjunct in a manner dangerous to patient

You must factually document your rationale for checking any of the above critical items on the reverse side of this form.

National Registry of Emergency Medical Technicians
Advanced Level Practical Examination

DYNAMIC CARDIOLOGY

Candidate: _____ Examiner: _____

Date: _____ Signature: _____

SET #_____

Level of Testing: □ NREMT-Intermediate/99   □ NREMT-Paramedic

Time Start:_____	Possible Points	Points Awarded
Takes or verbalizes infection control precautions	1	
Checks level of responsiveness	1	
Checks ABCs	1	
Initiates CPR when appropriate [verbally]	1	
Attaches ECG monitor in a timely fashion [patches, pads or paddles]	1	
Correctly interprets initial rhythm	1	
Appropriately manages initial rhythm	2	
Notes change in rhythm	1	
Checks patient condition to include pulse and, if appropriate, BP	1	
Correctly interprets second rhythm	1	
Appropriately manages second rhythm	2	
Notes change in rhythm	1	
Checks patient condition to include pulse and, if appropriate, BP	1	
Correctly interprets third rhythm	1	
Appropriately manages third rhythm	2	
Notes change in rhythm	1	
Checks patient condition to include pulse and, if appropriate, BP	1	
Correctly interprets fourth rhythm	1	
Appropriately manages fourth rhythm	2	
Orders high percentages of supplemental oxygen at proper times	1	
Time End: _____ **TOTAL**	24	

CRITICAL CRITERIA

_____ Failure to deliver any shock in a timely manner

_____ Failure to verify rhythm before delivering each shock

_____ Failure to ensure the safety of self and others [verbalizes "All clear" and observes]

_____ Inability to deliver DC shock [does not use machine properly]

_____ Failure to demonstrate acceptable shock sequence

_____ Failure to immediately order initiation or resumption of CPR when appropriate

_____ Failure to order correct management of airway [ET when appropriate]

_____ Failure to order administration of appropriate oxygen at proper time

_____ Failure to diagnose or treat 2 or more rhythms correctly

_____ Orders administration of an inappropriate drug or lethal dosage

_____ Failure to correctly diagnose or adequately treat v-fib, v-tach, or asystole

You must factually document your rationale for checking any of the above critical items on the reverse side of this form.

p306/8-003k

National Registry of Emergency Medical Technicians
Advanced Level Practical Examination

STATIC CARDIOLOGY

Candidate: _____   Examiner: _____

Date: _____   Signature: _____

SET #_____

Level of Testing: ☐ NREMT-Intermediate/99   ☐ NREMT-Paramedic

Note: No points for treatment may be awarded if the diagnosis is incorrect.
Only document incorrect responses in spaces provided.

Time Start:_____

	Possible Points	Points Awarded
STRIP #1 Diagnosis:	1	
Treatment:	2	
STRIP #2 Diagnosis:	1	
Treatment:	2	
STRIP #3 Diagnosis:	1	
Treatment:	2	
STRIP #4 Diagnosis:	1	
Treatment:	2	
TOTAL	12	

Time End: _____

p307/8-003k

INTRAVENOUS THERAPY

Candidate: _____ Examiner: _____

Date: _____ Signature: _____

Level of Testing: ❑ NREMT-Intermediate/85   ❑ NREMT-Intermediate/99   ❑ NREMT-Paramedic

Time Start: _____

	Possible Points	Points Awarded

Checks selected IV fluid for:
    -Proper fluid (1 point)
    -Clarity (1 point)
	2	

Selects appropriate catheter	1	
Selects proper administration set	1	
Connects IV tubing to the IV bag	1	
Prepares administration set [fills drip chamber and flushes tubing]	1	
Cuts or tears tape [at any time before venipuncture]	1	
Takes/verbalizes body substance isolation precautions [prior to venipuncture]	1	
Applies tourniquet	1	
Palpates suitable vein	1	
Cleanses site appropriately	1	

Performs venipuncture
    -Inserts stylette (1 point)
    -Notes or verbalizes flashback (1 point)
    -Occludes vein proximal to catheter (1 point)
    -Removes stylette (1 point)
    -Connects IV tubing to catheter (1 point)
	5	

Disposes/verbalizes disposal of needle in proper container	1	
Releases tourniquet	1	
Runs IV for a brief period to assure patent line	1	
Secures catheter [tapes securely or verbalizes]	1	
Adjusts flow rate as appropriate	1	

Time End: _____   **TOTAL**   21

CRITICAL CRITERIA

_____ Failure to establish a patent and properly adjusted IV within 6 minute time limit
_____ Failure to take or verbalize body substance isolation precautions prior to performing venipuncture
_____ Contaminates equipment or site without appropriately correcting situation
_____ Performs any improper technique resulting in the potential for uncontrolled hemorrhage, catheter shear, or air embolism
_____ Failure to successfully establish IV within 3 attempts during 6 minute time limit
_____ Failure to dispose/verbalize disposal of needle in proper container

NOTE: Check here (_____) if candidate did not establish a patent IV and do not evaluate IV Bolus Medications.

INTRAVENOUS BOLUS MEDICATIONS

Time Start: _____

Asks patient for known allergies	1	
Selects correct medication	1	
Assures correct concentration of drug	1	
Assembles prefilled syringe correctly and dispels air	1	
Continues body substance isolation precautions	1	
Cleanses injection site [Y-port or hub]	1	
Reaffirms medication	1	
Stops IV flow [pinches tubing or shuts off]	1	
Administers correct dose at proper push rate	1	
Disposes/verbalizes proper disposal of syringe and needle in proper container	1	
Flushes tubing [runs wide open for a brief period]	1	
Adjusts drip rate to TKO/KVO	1	
Verbalizes need to observe patient for desired effect/adverse side effects	1	

Time End: _____   **TOTAL**   13

CRITICAL CRITERIA

_____ Failure to begin administration of medication within 3 minute time limit
_____ Contaminates equipment or site without appropriately correcting situation
_____ Failure to adequately dispel air resulting in potential for air embolism
_____ Injects improper drug or dosage [wrong drug, incorrect amount, or pushes at inappropriate rate]
_____ Failure to flush IV tubing after injecting medication
_____ Recaps needle or failure to dispose/verbalize disposal of syringe and needle in proper container

You must factually document your rationale for checking any of the above critical items on the reverse side of this form.

p309/8-003k

National Registry of Emergency Medical Technicians
Advanced Level Practical Examination
ORAL STATION

Candidate: _____ Examiner: _____

Date: _____ Signature: _____

Scenario: _____

Time Start: _____

	Possible Points	Points Awarded
Scene Management		
Thoroughly assessed and took deliberate actions to control the scene	3	
Assessed the scene, identified potential hazards, did not put anyone in danger	2	
Incompletely assessed or managed the scene	1	
Did not assess or manage the scene	0	
Patient Assessment		
Completed an organized assessment and integrated findings to expand further assessment	3	
Completed initial, focused, and ongoing assessments	2	
Performed an incomplete or disorganized assessment	1	
Did not complete an initial assessment	0	
Patient Management		
Managed all aspects of the patient's condition and anticipated further needs	3	
Appropriately managed the patient's presenting condition	2	
Performed an incomplete or disorganized management	1	
Did not manage life-threatening conditions	0	
Interpersonal relations		
Established rapport and interacted in an organized, therapeutic manner	3	
Interacted and responded appropriately with patient, crew, and bystanders	2	
Used inappropriate communication techniques	1	
Demonstrated intolerance for patient, bystanders, and crew	0	
Integration (verbal report, field impression, and transport decision)		
Stated correct field impression and pathophysiological basis, provided succinct and accurate verbal report including social/psychological concerns, and considered alternate transport destinations	3	
Stated correct field impression, provided succinct and accurate verbal report, and appropriately stated transport decision	2	
Stated correct field impression, provided inappropriate verbal report or transport decision	1	
Stated incorrect field impression or did not provide verbal report	0	
TOTAL	15	

Time End: _____

Critical Criteria

_____ Failure to appropriately address any of the scenario's "Mandatory Actions"
_____ Performs or orders any harmful or dangerous action or intervention

You must factually document your rationale for checking any of the above critical items on the reverse side of this form.

p308/8-003k

PEDIATRIC (<2 yrs.) VENTILATORY MANAGEMENT

Candidate: _____ Examiner _____

Date: _____ Signature: _____

NOTE: If candidate elects to ventilate initially with BVM attached to reservoir and oxygen, full credit must be awarded for steps denoted by "**" so long as first ventilation is delivered within 30 seconds.

	Possible Points	Points Awarded
Takes or verbalizes body substance isolation precautions	1	
Opens the airway manually	1	
Elevates tongue, inserts simple adjunct [oropharyngeal or nasopharyngeal airway]	1	
NOTE: Examiner now informs candidate no gag reflex is present and patient accepts adjunct		
**Ventilates patient immediately with bag-valve-mask device unattached to oxygen	1	
**Ventilates patient with room air	1	
NOTE: Examiner now informs candidate that ventilation is being performed without difficulty and that pulse oximetry indicates the patient's blood oxygen saturation is 85%		
Attaches oxygen reservoir to bag-valve-mask device and connects to high flow oxygen regulator [12-15 L/minute]	1	
Ventilates patient at a rate of 12-20/minute and assures visible chest rise	1	
NOTE: After 30 seconds, examiner auscultates and reports breath sounds are present, equal bilaterally and medical direction has ordered intubation. The examiner must now take over ventilation.		
Directs assistant to pre-oxygenate patient	1	
Identifies/selects proper equipment for intubation	1	
Checks laryngoscope to assure operational with bulb tight	1	
NOTE: Examiner to remove OPA and move out of the way when candidate is prepared to intubate		
Places patient in neutral or sniffing position	1	
Inserts blade while displacing tongue	1	
Elevates mandible with laryngoscope	1	
Introduces ET tube and advances to proper depth	1	
Directs ventilation of patient	1	
Confirms proper placement by auscultation bilaterally over each lung and over epigastrium	1	
NOTE: Examiner to ask, "If you had proper placement, what should you expect to hear?"		
Secures ET tube [may be verbalized]	1	
TOTAL	17	

CRITICAL CRITERIA

_____ Failure to initiate ventilations within 30 seconds after applying gloves or interrupts ventilations for greater than 30 seconds at any time

_____ Failure to take or verbalize body substance isolation precautions

_____ Failure to pad under the torso to allow neutral head position or sniffing position

_____ Failure to voice and ultimately provide high oxygen concentrations [at least 85%]

_____ Failure to ventilate patient at a rate of 12-20/minute

_____ Failure to provide adequate volumes per breath [maximum 2 errors/minute permissible]

_____ Failure to pre-oxygenate patient prior to intubation

_____ Failure to successfully intubate within 3 attempts

_____ Uses gums as a fulcrum

_____ Failure to assure proper tube placement by auscultation bilaterally **and** over the epigastrium

_____ Inserts any adjunct in a manner dangerous to the patient

_____ Attempts to use any equipment not appropriate for the pediatric patient

You must factually document your rationale for checking any of the above critical items on the reverse side of this form.

National Registry of Emergency Medical Technicians
Advanced Level Practical Examination

PEDIATRIC INTRAOSSEOUS INFUSION

Candidate: _____ Examiner: _____

Date: _____ Signature: _____

Time Start:_____

	Possible Points	Points Awarded
Checks selected IV fluid for: 　　-Proper fluid (1 point) 　　-Clarity (1 point)	2	
Selects appropriate equipment to include: 　　-IO needle (1 point) 　　-Syringe (1 point) 　　-Saline (1 point) 　　-Extension set (1 point)	4	
Selects proper administration set	1	
Connects administration set to bag	1	
Prepares administration set [fills drip chamber and flushes tubing]	1	
Prepares syringe and extension tubing	1	
Cuts or tears tape [at any time before IO puncture]	1	
Takes or verbalizes body substance isolation precautions [prior to IO puncture]	1	
Identifies proper anatomical site for IO puncture	1	
Cleanses site appropriately	1	
Performs IO puncture: 　　-Stabilizes tibia (1 point) 　　-Inserts needle at proper angle (1 point) 　　-Advances needle with twisting motion until "pop" is felt (1 point) 　　-Unscrews cap and removes stylette from needle (1 point)	4	
Disposes of needle in proper container	1	
Attaches administration set to IO needle (with or without 3-way)	1	
Slowly injects saline to assure proper placement of needle	1	
Adjusts flow rate as appropriate	1	
Secures needle with tape and supports with bulky dressing	1	

Time End: _____ 　　　　　　　　　　　　**TOTAL** 23

CRITICAL CRITERIA
_____ Failure to establish a patent and properly adjusted IO line within the 6 minute time limit
_____ Failure to take or verbalize body substance isolation precautions prior to performing IO puncture
_____ Contaminates equipment or site without appropriately correcting situation
_____ Performs any improper technique resulting in the potential for air embolism
_____ Failure to assure correct needle placement
_____ Failure to successfully establish IO infusion within 2 attempts during 6 minute time limit
_____ Performing IO puncture in an unacceptable manner [improper site, incorrect needle angle, etc.]
_____ Failure to dispose of needle in proper container
_____ Orders or performs any dangerous or potentially harmful procedure

You must factually document your rationale for checking any of the above critical items on the reverse side of this form.

National Registry of Emergency Medical Technicians
Advanced Level Practical Examination

SPINAL IMMOBILIZATION (SEATED PATIENT)

Candidate: _____ Examiner: _____

Date: _____ Signature: _____

Time Start: _____	Possible Points	Points Awarded
Takes or verbalizes body substance isolation precautions	1	
Directs assistant to place/maintain head in the neutral, in-line position	1	
Directs assistant to maintain manual immobilization of the head	1	
Reassesses motor, sensory, and circulatory function in each extremity	1	
Applies appropriately sized extrication collar	1	
Positions the immobilization device behind the patient	1	
Secures the device to the patient's torso	1	
Evaluates torso fixation and adjusts as necessary	1	
Evaluates and pads behind the patient's head as necessary	1	
Secures the patient's head to the device	1	
Verbalizes moving the patient to a long backboard	1	
Reassesses motor, sensory, and circulatory function in each extremity	1	
Time End: _____ **TOTAL**	12	

CRITICAL CRITERIA

_____ Did not immediately direct or take manual immobilization of the head

_____ Did not properly apply appropriately sized cervical collar before ordering release of manual immobilization

_____ Released or ordered release of manual immobilization before it was maintained mechanically

_____ Manipulated or moved patient excessively causing potential spinal compromise

_____ Head immobilized to the device **before** device sufficiently secured to torso

_____ Device moves excessively up, down, left, or right on the patient's torso

_____ Head immobilization allows for excessive movement

_____ Torso fixation inhibits chest rise, resulting in respiratory compromise

_____ Upon completion of immobilization, head is not in a neutral, in-line position

_____ Did not reassess motor, sensory, and circulatory functions in each extremity after voicing immobilization to the long backboard

You must factually document your rationale for checking any of the above critical items on the reverse side of this form.

p311/8-003k

SPINAL IMMOBILIZATION (SUPINE PATIENT)

Candidate: _____ Examiner: _____

Date: _____ Signature: _____

	Possible Points	Points Awarded
Time Start: _____		
Takes or verbalizes body substance isolation precautions	1	
Directs assistant to place/maintain head in the neutral, in-line position	1	
Directs assistant to maintain manual immobilization of the head	1	
Reassesses motor, sensory, and circulatory function in each extremity	1	
Applies appropriately sized extrication collar	1	
Positions the immobilization device appropriately	1	
Directs movement of the patient onto the device without compromising the integrity of the spine	1	
Applies padding to voids between the torso and the device as necessary	1	
Immobilizes the patient's torso to the device	1	
Evaluates and pads behind the patient's head as necessary	1	
Immobilizes the patient's head to the device	1	
Secures the patient's legs to the device	1	
Secures the patient's arms to the device	1	
Reassesses motor, sensory, and circulatory function in each extremity	1	
Time End: _____ **TOTAL**	14	

CRITICAL CRITERIA

_____ Did not immediately direct or take manual immobilization of the head
_____ Did not properly apply appropriately sized cervical collar before ordering release of manual immobilization
_____ Released or ordered release of manual immobilization before it was maintained mechanically
_____ Manipulated or moved patient excessively causing potential spinal compromise
_____ Head immobilized to the device **before** device sufficiently secured to torso
_____ Patient moves excessively up, down, left, or right on the device
_____ Head immobilization allows for excessive movement
_____ Upon completion of immobilization, head is not in a neutral, in-line position
_____ Did not reassess motor, sensory, and circulatory functions in each extremity after voicing immobilization to the device

You must factually document your rationale for checking any of the above critical items on the reverse side of this form.

BLEEDING CONTROL/SHOCK MANAGEMENT

Candidate: _____ Examiner: _____

Date: _____ Signature: _____

Time Start:_____	Possible Points	Points Awarded
Takes or verbalizes body substance isolation precautions	1	
Applies direct pressure to the wound	1	
NOTE: The examiner must now inform the candidate that the wound continues to bleed.		
Applies tourniquet	1	
NOTE: The examiner must now inform the candidate that the patient is exhibiting signs and symptoms of hypoperfusion.		
Properly positions the patient	1	
Administers high concentration oxygen	1	
Initiates steps to prevent heat loss from the patient	1	
Indicates the need for immediate transportation	1	
Time End: _____	**TOTAL** 7	

CRITICAL CRITERIA

_____ Did not take or verbalize body substance isolation precautions
_____ Did not apply high concentration of oxygen
_____ Did not control hemorrhage using correct procedures in a timely manner
_____ Did not indicate the need for immediate transportation

You must factually document your rationale for checking any of the above critical items on the reverse side of this form.

SECTION III

ANSWERS
TO QUESTIONS

Chapter 1

Case Study

1. *What are the predictable injuries based on the mechanism of injury?*

   The scenario suggests that the driver was ejected from the motor vehicle. Following an up-and-over trajectory, the driver likely experienced head and neck injuries as his head struck the windshield and chest injuries as his body struck the steering wheel. Injuries following the ejection are a function of the trajectory and objects that the driver struck in flight.

2. *What modern safety equipment might have prevented these injuries?*

   Seat belts and airbags are used to restrain the driver in the vehicle. Safety glass in the windshield is another safety feature. Crumple zones and deforming bumpers also decrease the energy of the crash and thus decrease the likelihood of ejection.

3. *What is the most appropriate triage decision here?*

   Utilizing the American College of Surgeons Field Triage Criteria, the Paramedics should decide if the patient meets major trauma criteria. The first step in that decision tree is differentiating the physiologically stable patient from the unstable patient. Next, the Paramedic should use anatomical criteria to differentiate serious injuries from non-life-threatening injuries. Finally, the Paramedic should look at the mechanism of injury as a predictor of injury.

4. *Does this patient meet major trauma criteria?*

   Despite the apparent lack of information, this patient does meet major trauma criteria because he was ejected from a motor vehicle during a collision.

Practice Questions

Multiple Choice

1. c
2. a
3. c
4. b
5. a
6. b
7. a
8. a
9. a
10. a
11. a
12. c
13. d
14. c
15. d

Short Answer

16. Both trauma and infectious disease have demographic distributions, predictable seasonal patterns, epidemic episodes, and risk factors.

17. Triage is defined as the process of sorting patients according to their need and available resources.

18. Undertriage is failure to properly identify seriously ill and injured patients, whereas overtriage is misidentification of minor injuries and illnesses, giving them a higher priority than warranted.

19. By identifying the mechanism of injury, the Paramedic can apply her knowledge of kinematics and ascertain the predictable injury pattern.

20. Women tend to stab with an overhand motion going downward, whereas men tend to stab with an upward motion.

Fill in the Blank

21. excessive force

22. penetrating trauma

23. velocity, mass

24. lay down

25. soft body armor

Chapter 2

Case Study

Chief Concern

1. *What are some of the possible traumatic brain injuries that would be suspected based on the mechanism of injury?*

   Brain injuries can range from a mild soft-tissue injury, such as a concussion, to an extracerebral hemorrhage. However, the severity of the crash suggests the patient may have a more serious head injury, including subdural and epidural hematoma.

2. *Are any of these traumatic brain injuries potentially life-threatening conditions?*

   Extracerebral hemorrhages can create a space-occupying lesion, increasing intracranial pressure and leading to herniation syndromes.

History

1. *What is the most important element of the history for a trauma patient?*

   The most important element of the history of a trauma patient is the mechanism of injury, which should lead the Paramedic to a predictable injury pattern. However, if possible, the Paramedic should use the mnemonic SAMPLE and try to obtain a standard medical history.

2. *What* specific *elements of the history should the Paramedic obtain from this patient?*

   Specifically, in terms of traumatic brain injury, the Paramedic should ascertain if there is any loss of consciousness, headache, and neck pain. The Paramedic should also inquire about allergies, particularly to lidocaine (lidocaine is used prior to intubation). During the medication history, the Paramedic should focus on anticoagulants that may worsen intracranial hemorrhage as well as medications, such as beta blockers, that can prevent a protective response to increasing intracranial hemorrhage.

Examination

1. *What are the elements of the physical examination of a patient with suspected herniation syndrome?*

   Beyond the primary assessment, the Paramedic must focus on the patient's level of consciousness. Subtle changes in the level of consciousness may be the only initial indication of increasing intracranial pressure. The Paramedic should next focus on the breathing pattern for early changes, such as Cheyne–Stokes respiration, and vital signs, as well as pupillary changes (i.e., brisk to sluggish to fixed to dilated). These are all signs of increasing intracranial pressure.

2. *Why are vital signs a critical element in this examination?*

   The vital signs for a head-injured patient are opposite of those of a shock–trauma patient (i.e., the pulse is down and the blood pressure is up). However, it is important to prevent hypotension in the multitrauma patient who has had a traumatic brain injury.

Assessment

1. *What is the significance of the area impacted?*

   The area of impact (the temporoparietal area) is proximal to the pterion, the most common site of epidural hematoma. Trauma to the area can result in injury to the middle meningeal artery.

2. *What is the patient's prognosis?*

Although epidural bleeds make up only a small percentage of traumatic brain injuries (about 1% to 2 % of the total), they have a high associated mortality (up to 43%). Therefore, if the patient does have an epidural hematoma, the prognosis is poor and the injury is life-threatening.

Treatment

1. *What is the national standard of care of patients with suspected traumatic brain injury?*

The Paramedic's first priority is to stabilize and support the patient. The Paramedic should ensure proper oxygenation (to prevent hypoxia) and adequate blood glucose. She must also take measures to reverse hypoglycemia. It is also important to pay careful attention to the patient's vital signs. The therapeutic goal of fluid resuscitation is to maintain a mean arterial pressure of approximately 70 to 80 mmHg, slightly higher than normal, in order to compensate for increasing intracranial pressure.

2. *What are some of the patient-specific concerns and considerations that the Paramedic should consider when applying this plan of care that is intended to treat a broad patient population presenting with acute herniation syndrome?*

The Paramedic should be cautious about fluid resuscitation, as an unplanned fluid bolus can increase intracranial pressure. However, if the patient is hypotensive (e.g., secondary to internal hemorrhage), then the Paramedic should institute fluid resuscitation with the therapeutic goal of maintaining a mean arterial pressure of 70 to 80 mmHg. A single episode of hypotension has been related to a 50% mortality in head trauma patients.

Evaluation

1. *What are some of the predictable complications associated with acute herniation syndrome?*

The combativeness may be due to hypoglycemia (although this is unlikely), hypoxia, or even hypotension. However, as these conditions are being monitored, the likely explanation is a cingulate herniation, a form of transtentorial herniation.

2. *What are some of the predictable complications associated with the treatment of acute herniation syndromes?*

Hypothetically, hyperventilation reduces carbon dioxide and thereby causes vasoconstriction. This, in turn, slows the bleeding. However, hyperventilation is nonselective, meaning that it decreases perfusion to the entire brain, as well as to bleeding blood vessels. Eventually hyperventilation, and the subsequent pancerebral anoxia, can have a negative impact on the patient.

Disposition

1. *What is the most appropriate transport decision that will get the patient to definitive care?*

Patients with suspected traumatic brain injury should be transported to a trauma center where neurosurgeons are available. These cases are high priority.

2. *What are the advantages of transporting a patient with suspected acute herniation syndrome to these hospitals, even if that means bypassing other hospitals in the process?*

The treatment of choice for a patient with suspected transtentorial herniation is trephination performed by a neurosurgeon. These procedures are generally only carried out in a trauma center.

Practice Questions
Multiple Choice

1. d		6. b	
2. a		7. c	
3. b		8. c	
4. b		9. c	
5. a		10. c	

11. d

12. a

13. a

14. c

15. c

Short Answer

16. Traumatic brain injury is a traumatic insult to the brain capable of producing intellectual, emotional, social, and vocational changes.

17. The symptom pattern for a concussion may or may not include loss of consciousness, headache, perseverating, momentary disorientation, and possible retrograde amnesia.

18. The Monroe–Kellie hypothesis states that when two materials occupy the same confined space, an increase in one volume must result in a decrease of the other volume.

19. Hippus is a rapid alternating constriction and dilation to bright light, which is an early indication of herniation.

20. Signs of a basilar skull fracture are otorrhea and/or rhinorrhea, retroauricle hematoma (Battle's sign), and bilateral periorbital ecchymosis (Raccoon eyes).

Fill in the Blank

21. mass effect

22. 48, 72

23. lucid interval

24. mean arterial pressure (MAP), intracranial pressure (ICP)

25. Biot's

Chapter 3

Case Study

Chief Concern

1. *What are some of the possible facial injuries that would be suspected based on the mechanism of injury?*

   A multitude of facial injuries are possible including Le Fort fractures, orbital blowout fractures, and minor facial fractures, such as fractures of the nasal septum or zygoma. Dental trauma is also likely.

2. *Are any of these facial injuries potentially life-threatening conditions?*

   Of the potential injuries to the face, excluding loss of airway, the more problematic injuries may be injuries to the neck including laryngeal swelling and hematoma formation.

History

1. *What are the important elements of the history that the Paramedic should obtain?*

   In trauma, the mechanism of injury leads to a suspicion of the injuries. A structural beam to the head should lead the Paramedic to question the patient about loss of consciousness, headache, and other symptoms of a traumatic brain injury.

   As this patient may be destined to go to the operating room, the Paramedic should try to obtain as complete a SAMPLE history as possible.

2. *What additional elements of the history should the Paramedic obtain?*

   Part of the assessment of facial injuries includes the determination of any pain as well as an assessment of the sensory organs (i.e., loss of vision and hearing impairment).

Examination

1. *What are the elements of the physical examination of a patient with suspected Le Fort fractures?*

The examination of the patient with suspected neck and face trauma should be methodical. After completing an assessment for life-threatening injuries in the primary assessment, some Paramedics start at the top of the head and move downward, checking the facial bones and the pupils (including extraocular movements). Next, the Paramedic inspects the nasal bones, the oral pharynx, the posterior auricle, and the base of the skull (basilar skull fracture), then proceeds to thoroughly assess the structures within the next area. Other Paramedics prefer to start with the oropharynx and move outward in a concentric ring.

2. *Why would a cranial nerve exam be a critical element in this examination?*

Not only does cranial nerve involvement suggest traumatic brain injury, but loss of extraocular movements may indicate an orbital fracture, with accompanying retinal detachment, as well as facial fractures.

Assessment

1. *What is the significance of the patient's loss of vision?*

Orbital or blowout fractures often accompany Le Fort fractures. A subsequent consequence of a blowout fracture is retinal detachment, leading to a loss of vision.

2. *What is the patient's prognosis?*

Although concerns about loss of vision secondary to retinal detachment are high on the priority list, an underlying head injury and/or basilar skull fracture may be a more life-threatening condition.

Treatment

1. *What is the first priority in the care of patients with suspected midface fractures?*

Airway management is the number one priority in the care of the patient with a midface fracture. However, intubation may not be possible, secondary to distorted anatomy, nor desirable if the patient must be sedated with a tenuous airway. Use of blind airway devices may be indicated.

2. *What is the next priority in the care of patients with suspected midface fractures?*

After ensuring ventilation and adequate oxygenation, the Paramedic can focus on controlling hemorrhage where possible. Although it is not possible to bleed to death into the skull (the patient will die from transtentorial herniation first), it is possible to bleed to death from facial lacerations. Scalp lacerations are well-known for bleeding copiously.

Evaluation

1. *What are some of the predictable complications associated with midface fractures?*

Bleeding from Le Fort fractures can be significant and can lead to hypotension. This bleeding can be evident (i.e., visible externally), or it can be hidden as blood passes down the esophagus into the stomach. A predictable complication of swallowed blood is nausea and vomiting. Forceful vomiting in this case can dislodge stabilizing blood clots as well as worsen facial fractures.

2. *What are some of the predictable complications associated with the treatments for midface fractures?*

Although fluid resuscitation is in order for the hypotension secondary to the severe hemorrhage from the Le Fort II fracture, particularly since accompanying head injuries can often be worsened by hypotension, the fluid resuscitation must be balanced against the risk of increasing intracranial pressure.

Disposition

1. *What is the most appropriate transport decision that will get the patient to definitive care?*

As the patient has a significant risk for traumatic brain injury and spinal cord injury, as well as facial fractures, the patient should be transported to a trauma center.

2. *What are the advantages of transporting a patient with suspected midface fractures to these hospitals, even if that means bypassing other hospitals in the process?*

A trauma center will have the necessary specialists including a neurosurgeon, orthopedic surgeon, ENT surgeon, and ophthalmologist.

Practice Questions
Multiple Choice

1. a		9. c
2. c		10. d
3. d		11. b
4. c		12. d
5. c		13. d
6. c		14. c
7. d		15. d
8. a		

Short Answer

16. The two mechanisms suspected of causing orbital blowout fractures are the hydraulic theory and the force/buckling theory.

17. Mandibular fractures often occur in pairs because the mandible is a ring and rings tend to break in two places.

18. The Paramedic should suspect a rapidly expanding hematoma within the neck.

19. The three zones of neck injuries are Zone I, which is from the clavicle to the cricoid; Zone II, which is from the cricoid to the mandible; and Zone III, which is from the mandible to the base of the skull.

20. The paper bag effect occurs when the patient holds his breath, forcing air expelled by the compressed chest against the closed glottis. The result can be traumatic tracheal rupture and internal neck injury.

Fill in the Blank

21. tympanic membrane perforation

22. auricular hematoma

23. traumatic iritis

24. retinal detachment

25. René Le Fort

Chapter 4
Case Study
Chief Concern

1. *What are some of the possible medical causes of paralysis?*

The causes of paralysis are numerous. Starting at the origin, there can be a disconnect between the brain's motor centers and the body. This occurs in a stroke. Next, there can be problems in the nerve impulse transmission, specifically the spinal cord. Demyelinating diseases, such as multiple sclerosis, can interrupt spinal cord transmission. Finally, the signal can be interrupted at the neuromuscular junction. This is what occurs in neuromuscular diseases such as polio.

2. *What are some of the possible traumatic causes of paralysis?*

Partial or complete transection of the spinal cord, from either penetrating trauma or blunt trauma, can interrupt the signal from brain to muscle.

History

1. *What is the first element of the history that a Paramedic should obtain?*

First, the Paramedic should determine the mechanism of injury as well as the nature of the injury. Although not among the listed high-risk mechanisms of injury, this case presentation would qualify.

2. *What other elements of the history should the Paramedic try to obtain?*

Next, the Paramedic should try to obtain information on the patient's medical conditions (such as diabetes) and medications (such as anticoagulants) that may complicate his care. Another medical condition of concern is Down syndrome (atlanto-axial instability). Other medications of concern include those that prevent osteoporosis, such as biphosphates.

Examination

1. *What are the elements of the physical examination of a patient with suspected spinal cord syndrome?*

After ensuring manual stabilization of the cervical spine, the Paramedic should proceed to complete a primary assessment. Injuries to the cervical spine can cause decreased ventilation and/or loss of diaphragmatic control of breathing. Following the primary assessment, the Paramedic should proceed with a methodical head-to-toe assessment of the patient.

2. *Why is a dermatome-focused neurological examination a critical element in this examination?*

A dermatome-focused neurological examination is part of the detailed spinal examination. Establishing the level of paralysis and/or paresthesia can help the Paramedic estimate the level of spinal cord injury and possibly predict the complications that may occur.

Assessment

1. *What is the significance of the loss of feeling on one side of the body and loss of movement on the other side?*

The mixed clinical presentation for paralysis and paresthesia is suggestive of a partial cord transection. This presentation is consistent with Brown–Sequard syndrome.

2. *What diagnosis did the Paramedic announce to the patient?*

Although the Paramedic may be inclined to tell the patient that he has Brown–Sequard syndrome without further testing or seeing what develops with the passage of time, the Paramedic should limit the topic to spinal cord injury.

Treatment

1. *What is the national standard of care of patients with suspected spinal cord injury?*

Although a penetrating torso injury does not normally receive spinal immobilization, patients with a presentation of paralysis and/or paresthesia need to be immobilized to prevent secondary injury.

2. *What are some of the patient-specific concerns and considerations that the Paramedic should consider when applying this plan of care that is intended to treat a broad patient population presenting with spinal cord injury?*

In this case, the patient has an impaled object (i.e., the knife) that must be stabilized in the position that it was found until a surgeon can remove it. This alters standard practice, and makes maintaining neutral in-line stabilization of the spine difficult.

Evaluation

1. *Why were these spinal cord injury complications predictable?*

Although a partial cord injury is suspected, it is predictable that a complete cord transection could occur, secondary to handling, or that spinal swelling has further impacted distal function. The sudden loss of bladder control is consistent with spinal shock.

2. *What potentially life-threatening complication could occur because of spinal cord injury?*

The patient may experience neurogenic shock. Though rare, neurogenic shock is the result of loss of sympathetic vasoconstriction below the level of the spinal cord injury, resulting in massive vasodilation and a subsequent relative hypovolemia.

Disposition

1. *What is the most appropriate transport decision that will get the patient to definitive care?*

In most EMS systems, this patient will be transported to a trauma center, as the impaled object represents a potential life threat. In many systems, the patient with suspected spinal injury is transported to a trauma center.

2. *What are the advantages of transporting a patient with suspected spinal cord injury to these hospitals, even if that means bypassing other hospitals in the process?*

A trauma center will have a neurosurgeon available to assess and treat the patient. Recent experimental therapies using therapeutic hypothermia and steroids, for example, must be instituted almost immediately. Delays with transferring a patient might impact the effectiveness of these treatments.

Practice Questions
Multiple Choice

1. a
2. a
3. b
4. c
5. b
6. d
7. a
8. b

9. a
10. d
11. c
12. d
13. b
14. b
15. a

Short Answer

16. A "deadman's fall" can result in central cord syndrome, the most common of the partial cord syndromes. This syndrome results in upper body weakness.

17. Approximately 17% of patients with Trisomy 21 (Down syndrome) have atlanto-axial instability, an instability of the first and second cervical vertebrae caused by lax ligaments that can result in spinal cord transection. Spinal cord transection at C1/C2 can lead to tetraplegia, diaphragmatic paralysis, and death by respiratory arrest.

18. Sacral sparing is numbness in the perineal area and is suggestive of an incomplete spinal cord injury.

19. Taking a hold of the foot, the Paramedic firmly rakes the arch of the foot in a C shape. Flaring of the great toe is considered a positive Babinski. The Babinski reflex is an infantile reflex that diminishes when the child walks. Its return is suggestive of complete spinal cord transection.

20. Selective spinal immobilization is a form of medical triage in which spinal immobilization is withheld for those patients with minor trauma or those who are at low risk for spinal cord injury.

Fill in the Blank

21. quadriplegia

22. sensory, spinothalamic, motor, corticospinal

23. conus medullaris

24. SCIWORA

25. priapism

Chapter 5

Case Study

Chief Concern

1. *What are some of the possible causes of chest trauma?*

   Chest trauma can be divided into either blunt or penetrating trauma. Blunt trauma can be the result of falls and assaults, although motor vehicle collisions are still the number one cause. Causes of penetrating trauma can include knife wounds, gunshot wounds, or wounds created by other projectiles.

2. *How is trouble breathing related to chest trauma?*

   Life-threatening trauma to the chest can be divided into two categories: vascular or pulmonary. Pulmonary problems can be further divided into problems of ventilation (e.g., fractured ribs that alter the mechanics of breathing) or respirations (e.g., a pulmonary contusion that prevents aeration and oxygenation).

History

1. *What are the important elements of the history that a Paramedic should obtain?*

   The Paramedic should ascertain the mechanism of injury before proceeding with the medical history. Knowledge of the mechanism of injury can help the Paramedic determine the predictable injury pattern.

2. *What important medical history should also be obtained?*

   A history of pulmonary disease, such as chronic obstructive pulmonary disease, can have a dramatic impact on the mechanics of ventilation and pulmonary respiration.

Examination

1. *What are the elements of the physical examination of a patient with chest trauma?*

   Chest trauma has serious implications to the primary assessment. Therefore, problems encountered during the primary assessment should be addressed first. Next, the Paramedic should methodically assess the chest wall using a look, listen, and feel approach.

2. *Why is auscultation a critical element in this examination?*

   Auscultation of lung sounds reaffirms the passage of air into and out of the alveolus. Absent, diminished, or adventitious breath sounds indicate an alteration in respiration and the potential for hypoxia.

Assessment

1. *What is the significance of the patient's absent breath sounds?*

   Absent breath sounds in the apices may indicate a pneumothorax, as air rises, whereas absent breath sounds in the bases may indicate a hemothorax, as liquids settle.

2. *Does the patient lying supine affect the Paramedic's physical findings?*

   As air rises, breath sounds in the supine patient may not be impressive until the pneumothorax is in an advanced stage.

Treatment

1. *What is the national standard of care of patients with a sucking chest wound?*

   An occlusive dressing is usually placed over a sucking chest wound. Although some Paramedics place a three-sided dressing over a sucking chest wound, the utility of this dressing is questionable.

2. *What are alternative treatments for a sucking chest wound?*

   In some cases where there is a short transportation time, it may be acceptable to leave the wound uncovered, particularly if the Paramedic is watchful for signs of a tension pneumothorax. Alternatively, any occlusive dressing is acceptable. The Paramedic must monitor for signs of a tension pneumothorax and be prepared to "burp" the dressings (i.e., release a corner of the dressing to release the pressure, as needed). Some occlusive dressings are made with a tab which is intended to help the Paramedic burp the dressing.

Evaluation

1. *What are some of the predictable complications associated with simple pneumothorax?*

   The most ominous complication of a simple pneumothorax is development of a tension pneumothorax. This potentially life-threatening complication should be foremost in the Paramedic's mind.

2. *What are some of the predictable complications associated with the treatments for a tension pneumothorax?*

   Misplacement of the decompression under the rib can result in perforation of the costal artery or vein. Shallow needle insertion can result in failure to decompress the pneumothorax, whereas deep needle insertion can potentially puncture the heart and/or great vessels.

Disposition

1. *Are there any dangers associated with air medical evacuation?*

   Although changes in barometric pressures may increase the incidence of pneumothorax or the development of a tension pneumothorax, most air medical services purposely fly at lower altitudes to prevent these problems.

2. *What is the most appropriate transport decision that will get the patient to definitive care?*

   Patients with penetrating chest trauma should be transported to a trauma center where thoracic surgeons are prepared to care for the potentially life-threatening injuries.

Practice Questions
Multiple Choice

1. d
2. b
3. c
4. c
5. d
6. a
7. b
8. d
9. c
10. a
11. b
12. a
13. a
14. a
15. d

Short Answer

16. Although the fractured ribs of a flail chest are ominous, the presence of paradoxical motion demonstrates the alteration in mechanics of breathing that makes a flail chest problematic.

17. A diaphragmatic rupture, or diaphragmatic herniation, occurs when forces to the abdomen push abdominal contents into the chest cavity. The result is a functional ventilatory restriction.

18. Commotio cordis occurs when the heart is struck during a vulnerable period, leading to ventricular fibrillation.

19. Increased pressure in the chest, caused by accumulated air, results in decreased preload, tamponade of the heart, and kinking of the outflow tract, specifically the aorta. The combination of these three events culminates in hypotension.

20. A tension pneumothorax is a simple pneumothorax associated with hypotension. Along with all the symptoms of a simple pneumothorax, a tension pneumothorax may be associated with jugular venous distention, tracheal deviation, and muffled heart sounds.

Fill in the Blank

21. flail chest
22. diaphragmatic herniation
23. myocardial contusion
24. traumatic aortic disruptions
25. sucking chest wound

Chapter 6
Case Study
Chief Concern

1. *What potentially life-threatening injuries could occur from being kicked in the abdomen by a cow?*

   The list of potential internal injuries is long but can be broken down into injuries to solid organs (such as the liver and spleen), injuries to hollow organs (such as the intestines and bladder), and internal vascular injury.

2. *Which of these are the most life-threatening injuries?*

   Of these injuries, vascular injuries may be immediately life-threatening on-scene, whereas injuries to the solid organs may manifest during the course of patient care.

History

1. *What are the important elements of the history that a Paramedic should obtain?*

   The mechanism of injury is particularly important when assessing the extent of injury from trauma. If the patient is experiencing pain, then the OPQRST mnemonic is helpful in establishing the degree of injury. Conditions that often complicate trauma care included pre-existing chronic disease such as heart failure, lung disease, and so on, as well as certain medications such as anticoagulants and beta blockers.

2. *Why would the use of beta blockers be problematic?*

   The body's response to hemorrhage is the sympathetic nervous system. Beta blockers limit the heart's ability to respond to sympathetic stimulation and to mount a compensatory tachycardia in the face of lost volume (SV x HR = CO). Without an increase in heart rate to compensate for the hemorrhagic losses, the blood pressure falls.

Examination

1. *What are the elements of the physical examination of a patient with suspected internal abdominal hemorrhage?*

   After the primary assessment, the Paramedic should take a look, listen, and feel approach to the physical examination of the abdomen. The Paramedic should especially look for ecchymosis, as ecchymotic areas may indicate underlying organ injury. Similarly, the Paramedic should look for abdominal distention resulting from internal hemorrhage.

2. *Why is the fact that the patient's abdomen is distended of concern?*

   The abdomen can hold up to 3 liters of fluid before it may appear distended. As the average human body is estimated to contain between 5 to 7 liters, this fluid loss could represent life-threatening hypovolemia and result in decompensated shock.

Assessment

1. *What are the potential sources of bleeding?*

   Internal organs of the abdomen can be divided into solid and hollow organs. The solid organs, particularly the spleen and liver, carry the greatest risk for bleeding. The presence of point tenderness and deformity of the lower floating ribs should make the Paramedic suspicious of spleen and/or liver injury.

2. *What is the Paramedic's diagnosis?*

   Based on the mechanism of injury and patient presentation, the Paramedic can assume internal bleeding and should treat the patient for suspected hemorrhagic shock.

Treatment

1. *What is the national standard of care of patients with suspected abdominal injury?*

   As the patient with abdominal injury may compensate for an extended period of time, the Paramedic must have a high index of suspicion of internal injury even if the patient does not immediately present with symptoms of hemorrhagic shock.

2. *Is there any referred pain that would be suggestive of abdominal injury?*

Injuries to the spleen often refer pain to the right shoulder, and liver injuries refer pain to the left shoulder.

Evaluation

1. *What are some of the predictable complications associated with an internal abdominal bleeding patient?*

As the solid organs are encapsulated, blood can collect, effectively creating a tamponade effect. Although this initially contains and controls the bleeding, this effect is limited. Eventual rupture of the capsule, hours or days later, can lead to catastrophic hemorrhage.

2. *What are some of the predictable complications associated with the treatments for massive hemorrhage?*

The therapeutic goal of fluid resuscitation is to keep an adequate blood pressure to maintain cerebral perfusion without increasing the blood pressure to the point where established blood clots are dislodged and/or clotting factors are unnecessarily diluted.

Disposition

1. *What is the most appropriate transport decision that will get the patient to definitive care?*

Patients with blunt trauma and internal hemorrhage need to be cared for at a trauma center where vascular surgeons, as well as a blood bank, are available.

2. *What are some of the transportation considerations?*

In the rural setting, where a trauma center may be more than an hour away, rapid transportation via helicopter must be considered as part of the patient care plan early in the course of care.

Practice Questions
Multiple Choice

1. c
2. a
3. a
4. c
5. b
6. d
7. d
8. a
9. b
10. d
11. d
12. c
13. c
14. c
15. b

Short Answer

16. The abdominal cavity can hold up to 3 liters of blood or fluid without visible distention.

17. FAST is the Focused Abdominal Sonography in Trauma exam. Using ultrasound, Paramedics can look for free blood in the abdomen.

18. A shearing injury occurs to the liver when, with sudden deceleration, the ligamentum teres hepatis literally tears the liver in half.

19. Steering wheels and handlebars, focusing energy to the abdomen, are examples of blunt trauma that can cause pancreatic injury.

20. Solid organs such as the liver, spleen, pancreas, and kidneys can all refer pain.

Fill in the Blank

21. left

22. gross hematuria

23. subcapsular hematomas

24. solid

25. retroperitoneal hematoma.

Chapter 7
Case Study
Chief Concern

1. *What are some of the possible orthopaedic trauma injuries that can be expected in the appendicular skeleton if the patient follows the up-and-over pathway?*

   Starting at the shoulder girdle, drivers often lock wrists before a collision. This may result in wrist and shoulder injuries. Injury to the pelvic girdle depends on the pathway. If the patient follows the up-and-over pathway, then femur fractures resulting from impact with the steering column may occur.

2. *What are some of the possible orthopaedic trauma injuries that can be expected in the appendicular skeleton if the patient follows the down-and-under pathway?*

   If the patient follows the down-and-under pathway, and strikes the crash bar, then the patient may dislocate the knees and/or the hips.

History

1. *What are the important elements of the history that a Paramedic should obtain if the collision was truck versus car in the lateral impact?*

   The most important element in this history is the mechanism of injury. The effect of a lateral impact on the patient is dependent on the size of the other vehicle and the line of force. If the collision is truck versus car, the driver of the car may have an injury to the shoulder girdle.

2. *What are the important elements of the history if the collision was car versus truck in the lateral impact?*

   If the reverse occurred, then the driver of the truck may have an injury to the pelvic girdle. In every instance, the Paramedic needs to assess the point of impact and predict the lines of force.

Examination

1. *What are the elements of the physical examination of a patient with suspected pelvic fracture?*

   Following the primary assessment, the Paramedic should perform a head-to-toe secondary assessment for further injuries. It is imperative that the Paramedic, while exposing the patient's hips, maintains her dignity.

   First, the Paramedic should assess for an open pelvis fracture. If none is present, then the Paramedic should assess for hemorrhage from the vagina and/or rectum. Visible external bleeding is suggestive of a "hidden" open pelvis fracture.

2. *Why is it inappropriate to "spring the hips"?*

   Application of force along the iliac crests (i.e., "rocking or springing" the hips) not only is a poor indicator of pelvic fracture, but it can convert a closed pelvis fracture into an open-book fracture.

Assessment

1. *What diagnosis did the Paramedic announce to the patient?*

   Although a diagnosis of a pelvic fracture will need an X-ray to confirm, the Paramedic can report to the patient that she may have a pelvic injury.

2. *What are the possibilities of associated spinal injuries?*

The Paramedic should also suspect that the patient has associated lower lumbar and sacral injury.

Treatment

1. *What is the national standard of care of patients with suspected pelvic fractures?*

Pelvic fractures should be immobilized using one of three devices: the pelvic binder, the pelvic sling, or military anti-shock trousers. Any of these devices can create a circumferential pressure that will keep any pelvic fractures closed.

2. *Which of these devices would be useful if the patient developed hypotension secondary to internal hemorrhage from pelvic fractures?*

The military anti-shock trousers (MAST) have the added benefit of treating shock as well as maintaining pelvic compression.

Evaluation

1. *What are some of the predictable complications associated with pelvic fractures?*

A closed pelvic fracture can become an open pelvic fracture, which can bleed as much as 4 liters of blood into the pelvis, placing the patient into profound hemorrhagic shock.

2. *What are some of the predictable complications associated with the treatments for sustained pelvic fractures?*

Like all instances of internal bleeding in trauma, the Paramedic must walk the fine line during fluid resuscitation between maintaining cerebral perfusion and not increasing bleeding. The best marker of minimally acceptable cerebral perfusion may be the patient's level of consciousness.

Disposition

1. *What is the most appropriate transport decision that will get the patient to definitive care?*

With a major mechanism of injury, unstable vital signs, and a potential pelvic fracture, the patient meets the national trauma triage criteria for transportation to a trauma center.

2. *What services does this patient need?*

Blood loss from a pelvic fracture can be impressive. Many patients will need a blood transfusion as well as immediate surgery to stabilize the fractures and prevent further bleeding. These services are available at a trauma center.

Practice Questions
Multiple Choice

1. d	9. a
2. a	10. a
3. d	11. b
4. a	12. d
5. a	13. d
6. b	14. b
7. c	15. a
8. a	

Short Answer

16. The common complication of a navicular/scaphoid fracture is avascular necrosis. This is owed to the single blood supply to the bone, which when fractured leaves one-half of the bone without a blood supply.

17. Shin splints (i.e., medial tibial stress syndrome) is the result of inflammation of the peroneal tendon that causes pain over the lower half of the anterior shin and can lead to a stress fracture. Shin splints can occur with pes planus (flat feet).

18. FACTS is a mnemonic for fracture assessment: function, arterial pulses, capillary refill, temperature, and sensation.

19. RICE is a mnemonic for fracture treatment: rest, ice, compression, and elevation.

20. Compartment syndrome is a reperfusion injury that is caused by pressure buildup in a limb secondary to either compressive external force or obstruction to venous outflow.

Fill in the Blank

21. biomechanics

22. elastic, plastic

23. shoulder impingement syndrome

24. dislocation, subluxation

25. short arm volar

Chapter 8

Case Study

Chief Concern

1. *What are some of the possible soft-tissue injuries that the Paramedic would suspect based on the mechanism of injury?*

   Dog bites can be particularly problematic. These animals can create tremendous crushing pressures with their jaws, snapping bones as well as gashing flesh. Therefore, the patient may have soft-tissue injuries, including punctures and lacerations, as well as neuromuscular damage and even facial fractures.

2. *Are any of these soft-tissue injuries potentially life-threatening conditions?*

   As dogs, like all carnivores, kill by strangulation, the Paramedic should carefully examine the patient's throat, specifically the trachea, for injury.

History

1. *What are the important elements of the history that a Paramedic should obtain?*

   The mechanism of injury is the first consideration. Although a toddler would not be expected to be on many medications, the Paramedic should nonetheless obtain a careful SAMPLE history, focusing on medications that can impair healing, such as corticosteroids, anticoagulants, chemotherapy, and NSAIDs, as well as debilitating health conditions, such as COPD, diabetes, and immunosuppression.

2. *What are the confounding factors for wound healing?*

   Two confounding factors for wound healing are tobacco smoking and malnutrition. Tobacco smoke contains carbon monoxide as well as nicotine, a potent vasoconstrictor. Poor nutrition, particularly a diet lacking in vitamin C, vitamin A, and zinc, can cause poor wound healing.

Examination

1. *What are the elements of the physical examination for soft-tissue injury?*

   Systematically, and using DCAP BTLS, the Paramedic should examine the patient's scalp, face, and neck, as well as the upper extremities, as these are the most commonly bitten areas.

2. *What are the descriptions of the wounds?*

There may be superficial to full thickness lacerations as well as punctures. Avulsions, either partial or complete, of the ears and nose are not uncommon. All wounds should be carefully examined with the idea that these may be open fractures.

Assessment

1. *What is the importance of making a determination of the type of wound?*

Gross wounds are either bleeding or nonbleeding and either clean or dirty. In this case, the wounds appear to be bleeding (though not vigorously) and are considered dirty (dog saliva has numerous pathogens).

2. *What is the prognostic implication?*

Although minor bleeding can actually help cleanse a wound of pathogens, moderate to severe bleeding, particularly of the vascular scalp and face, can be a life-threatening condition if not controlled. Owed to the nature of the injury (i.e., dog bites), these wounds will be lacerations that will require extensive decontamination, debridement, and suturing.

Treatment

1. *What is the national standard of care of patients with soft-tissue injuries?*

The first priority in wound care is to stop the bleeding. In many cases, the bleeding stops spontaneously. However, if bleeding persists the Paramedic may need to apply a dressing. In this case the bleeding, while impressive, is minor to moderate and controlled with simple dressings.

2. *Beyond initial first aid, what other care can be provided?*

If time permits, the Paramedic can attempt decontamination and irrigation.

Evaluation

1. *What are some of the predictable complications associated with dog bites?*

Although rabies is one of the over 64 pathogens identified in dog and cat saliva, it is more likely that another, more common infectious agent will be problematic rather than rabies.

2. *What immunizations might the child receive?*

The child will likely receive a tetanus shot to ensure prophylaxis.

Disposition

1. *What is the most appropriate transport decision that will get the patient to definitive care?*

Although most hospitals are capable of treating facial lacerations, the presence of the "step off" in the scalp wound, suggestive of an open cranial vault, elevates the severity of the patient's wounds and mandates trauma center care.

2. *What are some of the transportation considerations?*

Although the wounds are gruesome, the Paramedic needs to stay focused on the potential for a head injury and monitor the child for signs of increasing intracranial pressure.

Practice Questions
Multiple Choice

1. a
2. a
3. a
4. d
5. c

6. b
7. c
8. d
9. d
10. b

11. b

12. a

13. d

14. a

15. c

Short Answer

16. Primary wound healing occurs when the wound edges are clear and closely approximated, whereas secondary wound healing is delayed, involves scab formation, and eventually leads to scar formation.

17. Death on-scene from a crush injury is due to the release of potassium during traumatic rhabdomyolysis. Death days later is from acute renal failure from traumatic rhabdomyolysis.

18. The Mangled Extremity Severity Score (MESS) is a field score that determines the need for amputation. MESS takes into account skeletal/ soft-tissue injury, limb ischemia, shock, and age—all values that are obtainable in the field.

19. Topical antibiotics work on the antibacterial effect of precious metals, particularly silver and iodine.

20. A bioengineered skin equivalent is a human skin substitute that consists of dermal cells seeded into a bovine collagen matrix.

Fill in the Blank

21. hypertrophic, keloid

22. static tension, dynamic tension

23. bandage, dressing

24. Braden risk assessment scale

25. crush, reperfusion

Chapter 9

Case Study

Chief Concern

1. *What is anhydrous ammonia?*

Anhydrous ammonia is a colorless gas with a pungent smell. It is used in household oven and drain cleaners, and farmers use it for fertilizer. Anhydrous ammonia is an alkali that is readily absorbed into the skin.

2. *Why is anhydrous ammonia stolen?*

Anhydrous ammonia is one of the key ingredients in the "Nazi" method of making methamphetamine. It is readily available on farms and often stolen, as farms have minimal security and a small police presence.

History

1. *What are the important elements of the history that a Paramedic should obtain?*

After ensuring scene safety, anhydrous ammonia forms a cloud, is lighter than air, and tends to dissipate rapidly. The Paramedic should try to ascertain the time of the exposure as well as the length of the exposure, in terms of time. Although chemical meters can determine the concentration of anhydrous ammonia, direct contact with the escaping gas is likely to be greater than 1,000 ppm.

2. *What is the symptom pattern associated with exposure to anhydrous ammonia?*

Inhaled anhydrous ammonia creates an exothermic reaction in the airways. These burns will result in cough, wheeze, bronchospasm, and/or laryngospasm. Swelling of both the upper and lower airways will lead to profound hypoxia.

Examination

1. *What are the elements of the physical examination of a patient with suspected toxic exposure?*

The organs sensitive to anhydrous ammonia exposure are the skin, the eyes, and the lungs. Therefore, the physical examination focuses on these three organs.

2. *Why is a respiratory examination a critical element in this examination?*

Anhydrous ammonia burns the airway, causing a reactive airway. It is critical for the Paramedic to obtain a baseline and monitor airway patency throughout the duration of patient care.

Assessment

1. *What is the assessment of the patient's condition?*

This patient has multiple exposures (i.e., topical as well as inhalation) which complicate the patient's care. A physician may best guide complex care under these circumstances.

2. *What are the initial priorities of care based on the Paramedic's assessment?*

In cases of suspected poisoning, the Paramedic should, at a minimum, prevent hypoxia, hypoglycemia, and hypoperfusion, if possible.

Treatment

1. *What is the initial care of patients with exposure to anhydrous ammonia?*

Massive quantities of water are used to decontaminate the patient whose skin is exposed to anhydrous ammonia. If the eyes are exposed, then a Morgan lens can help to irrigate the eyes. It is important to remove the patient's contact lens, if worn, as the lens can trap ammonia underneath it. The skin and eye irrigation should go on for at least 20 minutes. However, the Paramedic must understand that, even when the surface contaminants are washed away, the ammonia continues to burn deeper under the skin, making this a full thickness wound.

2. *What is the focus of care of patients with exposure to anhydrous ammonia?*

Treatment for inhalation of anhydrous ammonia focuses on supportive care. In mild cases, the application of continuous positive airway pressure (CPAP) may be beneficial. However, the Paramedic must be prepared to assist ventilations with a bag-mask assembly, preferably with positive end-expiratory pressure (PEEP). In some cases, it may be necessary to intubate the patient to ensure a patent airway. If so, a larger-than-normal endotracheal tube is used to prevent plugging by sloughing tissue.

Evaluation

1. *What are the visible effects seen with a topical exposure to anhydrous ammonia?*

Topical exposure to anhydrous ammonia will leave a gray–yellow tinged burn in most cases; in this case, the anhydrous ammonia has been dyed pink.

2. *What are the effects of topical exposure to anhydrous ammonia that are not visible?*

As the anhydrous ammonia couples with water, making ammonium hydroxide, the tissues undergo liquefaction necrosis. The anhydrous ammonia continues to cause liquefaction necrosis until the hydroxyl ions are exhausted. As a result, the burn on the surface is only a small part of the deeper injury, analogous to seeing only the tip of the iceberg.

Disposition

1. *What is the most appropriate transport decision that will get the patient to definitive care?*

The exposed patient should be transported to a hospital equipped to handle hazardous materials exposure.

2. *Why is the appropriate transportation decision important?*

Although the antidotes for anhydrous ammonia exposure are common, the concern is bringing a contaminated patient into an emergency department that is not equipped to handle the patient, potentially exposing the staff and patients alike.

Practice Questions

Multiple Choice

1. c
2. d
3. c
4. a
5. b
6. a
7. b
8. a

9. c
10. d
11. c
12. a
13. a
14. d
15. c

Short Answer

16. Used for a circumferential burn, an emergency escharotomy is a surgical incision generally made in parallel lines along the plane of the burn patient's skin to allow expansion.

17. Signs of smoke inhalation include carbonaceous sputum, singed vibrissae, and stridor.

18. A chemical precursor to vitamin B12, hydroxocobalamin works competitively with hemoglobin for cyanide and binds harmlessly with it to be excreted in the urine.

19. Fluid creep is the result of early overresuscitation that leads to increased burn edema formation, abdominal compartment syndrome, and acute respiratory distress syndrome.

20. The Parkland formula is 4 mL of fluid for every kilogram weight times the body surface area burned. One-half is to be given in the first eight hours.

Fill in the Blank

21. coagulation
22. coagulation, liquefaction
23. resistor

24. Curling's ulcer
25. Morgan lens

Chapter 10

Case Study

Chief Concern

1. *What are some of the potentially life-threatening injuries that Dwayne sustained?*

   As children tend to fall head first, the most likely injury is a head injury. The head injury is likely to be accompanied by a spinal injury as well.

2. *What other secondary injuries could the child have sustained?*

   As the child fell, he may have struck branches on the way down that caused fractures and bruising.

History

1. *What are the important elements of the history that a Paramedic should obtain?*

   After obtaining the history of the present illness (i.e., the mechanism of injury), the Paramedic should ascertain the presence and location of any pain as well as loss of consciousness and paresthesia/paralysis.

2. *What additional information would be helpful?*

Considering the mechanism of injury, the potential exists that the child may go to the operating room. Therefore, the Paramedic should list any medical conditions and medications, as well as the patient's last meal.

Examination

1. *What are the elements of the physical examination of a pediatric trauma patient?*

The elements of the physical examination of the pediatric trauma patient are no different than the physical examination elements for an adult. However, the Paramedic should make efforts to preserve the modesty of these patients when possible.

2. *Why is a cranial nerve exam a critical element in this examination?*

Head injury is the number one cause of accidental death in this age population. A cranial nerve exam will help the Paramedic to establish a baseline as well as demonstrate any subtle neurological deficits.

Assessment

1. *What diagnosis did the Paramedic announce to the patient's mother?*

Based on the patient's presentation, it is accurate for the Paramedic to tell the mother that her son may have sustained a head injury secondary to the fall and that a head injury from a fall for a boy this age is not unusual.

2. *Based on the patient's age, is it appropriate to discuss the diagnosis with the patient?*

Although a 9-year-old may understand abstract concepts such as traumatic brain injury, the Paramedic must convey, in concrete terms, the nature of the injury and what the child can expect to occur next.

Treatment

1. *What is the national standard of care of patients with suspected traumatic brain injury?*

The key to treatment of the suspected pediatric brain injury is to maintain adequate oxygenation as well as ventilation. As is the case with every trauma patient, the Paramedic must maintain a secure airway as well as adequate blood pressure.

2. *How should this patient be positioned on the stretcher?*

In this case (a suspected head injury), the head of the stretcher should be elevated approximately 15 to 20 degrees to help with cerebral drainage and to help prevent the buildup of pressure within the skull.

Evaluation

1. *What are some of the predictable complications associated with pediatric chest trauma?*

In this case, the Paramedic should suspect both a pneumothorax and a liver/splenic injury. By striking branches on the way down, the patient may have struck his chest, collapsing a lung, without leaving the traditional signs of a fractured rib. This is because the child's ribs are pliable and spring back.

2. *What are some other predictable complications based on the mechanism of injury?*

The child may have struck his false ribs, lacerating the liver or spleen in the process. The membranes of the spleen and liver can temporarily cause a tamponade of the bleeding, preventing signs of hemorrhage and hypoperfusion.

Disposition

1. *Does Dwayne's mechanism of injury meet major trauma criteria?*

A fall of two to three times the patient's height makes this pediatric patient eligible for major trauma criteria. Furthermore, the suspected presence of a traumatic brain injury, with a Glasgow Coma Scale less than 14, coupled with the tension pneumothorax makes this boy a candidate for a pediatric trauma center.

2. *What is the most appropriate transport decision that will get the patient to definitive care?*

Owing to the potential lethality of the head injury, coupled with the pneumothorax, this patient is high priority and should be transported emergently to the closest pediatric trauma center.

Practice Questions

Multiple Choice

1. c
2. d
3. d
4. b
5. b
6. d
7. a
8. a
9. d
10. a
11. d
12. b
13. c
14. b
15. a

Short Answer

16. In a SCIWORA, the patient exhibits signs and symptoms that are typical of a spinal cord injury, even though X-rays or CT scans performed in the emergency department are normal. SCIWORA stands for spinal cord injury without obvious radiographic abnormality.

17. A stinger results from the stretching of nerves and is a transient neurologic symptom that occurs at the time of injury and resolves after a short period of time.

18. A blunt force applied to the sternum and transmitted to the heart, in some cases, may cause the equivalent of an R on T phenomenon, sending the child into ventricular tachycardia, ventricular fibrillation, or torsades de pointes. This is called commotio cordis.

19. Greenstick fractures occur when the force applied to the bone causes one side of the cortex to break while the other side bends or deforms.

20. Buckle fractures typically occur in younger children when the force has been applied as an axial load to the extremity.

Fill in the Blank

21. post concussive seizures
22. SCIWORA
23. commotio cordis
24. greenstick
25. Salter–Harris

Chapter 11

Case Study

1. *What are some of the possible life-threatening injuries that would be suspected based on the mechanism of injury?*

   The most obvious injuries would be tracheal damage, with subsequent loss of the airway and a cervical spine injury. The patient may have suffocated as a result of a crushed throat or a spinal cord injury at the level of C3, C4, and C5, the nerves that innervate the diaphragm.

2. *What else should the Paramedic suspect?*

   The Paramedic should also suspect ingestion of alcohol or other intoxicants. These ingestions may complicate the picture; for example, a benzodiazepine and alcohol may be causing respiratory depression as well.

3. *What is the most appropriate transport decision that will get the patient to definitive care?*

   As the patient is physiologically unstable and suffered a trauma, it is prudent to transport the patient to a trauma center for further evaluation, particularly for the coma.

4. *What are some of the transportation considerations?*

   Although speed is important, spinal stabilization is also important. Even ligamentous injury to the neck can destabilize the spinal column.

Practice Questions
Multiple Choice

1. b
2. a
3. a
4. d
5. d
6. d
7. b
8. d

9. a
10. b
11. d
12. c
13. c
14. c
15. a

Short Answer

16. Nitrogen washout, the replacement of nitrogen with oxygen, provides an oxygen reservoir to provide a time buffer during airway management procedures.

17. Permissive hypotension permits more controlled fluid resuscitation using physiologic measures to determine the need for administration of additional fluid.

18. A blood pressure cuff inflated 20 to 30 mmHg above the patient's systolic blood pressure can be used as a tourniquet to gain control of bleeding. Most blood pressure cuffs, however, are not able to maintain a constant pressure for an extended period of time and will likely need to be reinflated.

19. The sympathetic nervous system utilizes the spinal cord to distribute nerves. If the spinal cord is cut, then sympathetic spinal nerves cannot stimulate vasoconstriction, leading to neurogenic shock.

20. Basilar skull fracture is a contraindication to nasal intubation of the trauma patient.

Fill in the Blank

21. baroreceptors
22. Heimlich valve
23. permissive hypotension.

24. two, supraglottic airway
25. hematopoietic

Chapter 12
Case Study
Chief Concern

1. *What are some of the possible causes of the patient's syncope?*

   Assuming that the syncope and the heat wave are related, the patient's syncope may be from heat syncope, orthostatic hypotension (secondary to heat exhaustion), or heatstroke.

2. *Of these possibilities, which is potentially a life-threatening condition?*

   Heatstroke can lead to coma and death within hours.

History

1. *What are the important elements of the history that a Paramedic should obtain?*

The first element of the history is to identify if the patient is one of the populations at risk. Of course, the Paramedic should ascertain all the circumstances surrounding the syncope. Was the patient standing, sitting, or did he quickly get up? Was the patient on a ladder and did the patient fall? Did the patient treat himself and, if so, how?

Next, the Paramedic should ascertain if the event occurred during exertion, if the worker is new to the job, and if the patient is on any medications that would interfere with his ability to dissipate heat. A complete SAMPLE history, particularly of last oral intake, is important.

2. *What medications interfere with a person's ability to dissipate heat?*

The groups of medications that can make a person prone to heat illness can be broken down into three categories. The first category is stimulants such as sympathomimetics including cocaine and methamphetamines. The second category is those medications that interfere with sweating. These include anticholinergic-like medications such as antihistamines and antipsychotics, specifically neuroleptics such as haloperidol or chlorpromazine. The last category of medications consists of those that impair the cardiovascular response, such as beta blockers and diuretics.

Examination

1. *What are the elements of the physical examination of a patient with suspected heatstroke?*

As it is difficult to obtain a core temperature in the field, the Paramedic must rely on physical findings. The first sign of compensation is the profound tachycardia that accompanies the vasodilation. Although the blood pressure may be normal to low, the Paramedic must keep an eye on the widening pulse pressure that proceeds cardiovascular collapse.

2. *Why is a 12-lead ECG a critical element in this examination?*

Although vessel-related myocardial ischemia related to the tachycardia is possible, changes in the 12-lead ECG, specifically global ST elevations, are suggestive of an extracardiac stress that is causing myocardial ischemia.

Assessment

1. *What diagnosis did the Paramedic announce?*

Despite the presence of sweat, the diagnosis is hyperthermia, or heat illness, and suspected heatstroke.

2. *What was the key element of this diagnosis?*

The diagnosis is made, in part, due to the patient's altered mental status.

Treatment

1. *What is the national standard of care of patients with suspected heat illness?*

The key to patient survival in heatstroke is to cool the patient as rapidly as possible. After the assurance of a patent airway and administration of high-flow, high-concentration oxygen, the Paramedic should focus on means to cool the patient including strategic ice packing, evaporative methods, and ice water towels, if available.

2. *What is the therapeutic goal of cooling the patient?*

The patient should be cooled aggressively until he is about 101°F (38°C).

Evaluation

1. *What are some of the predictable complications associated with hyperthermia?*

Seizures, secondary to increased intracranial pressure, are a predictable complication of heatstroke that compound the problem tenfold by creating more heat. It is imperative that the seizures be stopped, and the patient treated for hypoxia, hypercarbia, hypotension, and hypoglycemia. The use of normal saline may be effective in treating the hyponatremia as well.

2. *What are some of the predictable complications associated with the complications of hyperthermia?*

Vigorous seizure activity during heatstroke can cause a breakdown of muscle and subsequent rhabdomyolysis. It may be necessary to administer sodium bicarbonate and/or fluid bolus to prevent the rhabdomyolysis.

Disposition

1. *What is the most appropriate transport decision that will get the patient to definitive care?*

This patient is critically ill and needs the services of an intensive care unit. Most full-service hospitals should be capable of providing care.

2. *What are some of the transportation considerations?*

While en route to the hospital, it is important for the Paramedic to call ahead. It will be important to continue the cooling upon arrival. Depending on the hospital, the emergency physician may consider the use of extracorporeal membrane oxygenation (ECMO), in which case specialists will need to be called in.

Practice Questions
Multiple Choice

1. a
2. d
3. d
4. a
5. a
6. a
7. c
8. d

9. d
10. d
11. c
12. a
13. d
14. a
15. c

Short Answer

16. Heat syncope occurs when as much as 3.8 liters of blood is shunted to the skin for cooling and thereby creates systemic hypotension.

17. Heatstroke has a triple impact on oxygenation. To begin, increased temperatures have a dramatic effect on the oxyhemoglobin curve, causing a rightward shift. Coupled with a change in red blood cell morphology, red blood cells become spherical at high temperature, and hypoxia ensues. A higher partial pressure of oxygen, via high-flow, high-concentration oxygen, is needed to treat the hypoxemia. In many cases, high-flow, high-concentration oxygen will not be enough. During heatstroke, marked acidosis occurs secondary to cellular dysfunction and further shifts the oxyhemoglobin curve to the right. This metabolic acidosis is evidenced by a marked increase in end-tidal carbon dioxide.

18. One evaporative technique for cooling the body has the Paramedic gently spray a cool mist, at about 60°F (15°C), over the patient. This water should be cooler than tepid or lukewarm water. The mist should moisten the skin but not be allowed to drip, as heat loss is greatest with evaporation. To speed evaporation, the Paramedic can use a high-powered fan to circulate air over the patient.

19. Rhabdomyolysis occurs as a result of vigorous exercise that injures skeletal muscle. That, in turn, releases myoglobin that clogs the kidneys and can cause acute renal failure.

20. Early signs of hyponatremia include increased thirst, muscle cramps, lethargy, and skeletal muscle spasms. The most common symptoms, in one study, were mental status changes, emesis, and nausea. These symptoms are all consistent with exertional heatstroke.

Fill in the Blank

21. thermolysis

22. heat index

23. dilutional hyponatremia

24. heat syncope

25. anhydrosis

Chapter 13

Case Study

Chief Concern

1. *What problems might the skier be experiencing?*

   Barring any other unmentioned medical conditions or trauma, the case suggests the patient may be suffering from cold-related illness.

2. *What factors may have led to this problem?*

   The most damaging factor is that the skiers have become wet, from sweat. Without insulation, the moisture undoubtedly wicked heat from the woman's body, causing hypothermia

History

1. *What are the important elements of the history that a Paramedic should obtain?*

   The story explains the mechanism of injury, a cold day with prolonged exposure to the elements. However, this information alone is not sufficient. The Paramedic should inquire about other medical conditions that could diminish the patient's ability to respond to cold stress. Conditions such as endocrine disorders (hypothyroidism) or certain medications (beta blockers) can impair a patient's ability to respond to cold stress.

2. *What role does age play in the problem of cold illness?*

   With diminished subcutaneous fat, the elderly cannot retain heat. These diminished fat reserves, coupled with poorer digestive function, can lead to malnutrition. As a result, the elderly may not have the energy to sustain shivering. Under the broad rubric of diminished physiologic capacity, the elderly are generally more prone to cold illness than younger people.

Examination

1. *What are the elements of the physical examination of a patient with suspected cold-related illness?*

   Beyond the standard primary assessment and vital signs, the Paramedic should assess the patient for shivering as well as a temperature, if possible.

2. *Why should a careful neurological examination be performed?*

   As a core temperature is hard to obtain in the field, the Paramedic must focus on a neurological examination to assess the patient's degree of cold-illness impairment. Signs of loss of fine motor skills include mumbling and stumbling. Pupils may be sluggish, dilated, and then fixed, with each change indicating a worsening condition.

Assessment

1. *What level of hypothermia is this patient experiencing?*

   Based on the history and physical examination, the patient appears to still be in mild hypothermia, as shown by the shivering, loss of fine motor coordination, and impaired judgment.

2. *What key finding suggests that the patient has progressed in her illness?*

   The key factor between mild and more severe hypothermia is the presence or absence of shivering.

Treatment

1. *What is the national standard of care of patients with suspected mild hypothermia?*

   Patients with mild hypothermia should be disrobed of wet clothing and covered with dry (and preferably warmed) blankets. Most importantly, however, they must be removed from the cold.

2. *What are some of the patient-specific concerns and considerations that the Paramedic should consider when applying this plan of care that is intended to treat a broad patient population presenting with mild hypothermia?*

   Although intravenous access is desirable, it is often difficult to obtain due to vasoconstriction. Similarly, although an ECG is desirable, it is often difficult to obtain because the cold skin fails to warm the electrode gel in order to form the electrode "bridge."

Evaluation

1. *What could have led to this event?*

   Exhausted from skiing, Saniyah probably had minimal glycogen stored to begin with and now has used up all of her immediately available energy, leading to a glycogen debt. Therefore, she lacks the ability to passively rewarm.

2. *What would be the treatment for this change to moderate hypothermia?*

   The Paramedic should start active external rewarming including use of heat lamps, covered heat packs, and the like. The Paramedic should also carefully monitor the patient's mental status. Washout of cold blood from the extremities could lower the patient's core temperature (i.e., after drop phenomena) and induce severe hypothermia.

Disposition

1. *What is the most appropriate transport decision that will get the patient to definitive care?*

   Most cases of mild to moderate hypothermia can be handled locally. However, cases of severe hypothermia should be transported to hospitals capable of extracorporeal core rewarming.

2. *What are some of the transportation considerations?*

   Patients with moderate to severe hypothermia must be handled carefully. Rough handling, including rough roads, can cause the fragile heart to go into ventricular fibrillation.

Practice Questions
Multiple Choice

1. a
2. d
3. d
4. a
5. a
6. d
7. a
8. a
9. c
10. c
11. c
12. a
13. b
14. b
15. a

Short Answer

16. Cold diuresis develops when shunted blood engorges the kidneys, leading to increased urine formation and diuresis.

17. Trench foot develops when a foot is continuously immersed in less than body temperature water.

18. The "umbles," signs of mild hypothermia, refer to stumble, mumble, fumble, and grumble.

19. In the after drop phenomenon, warmth applied to cold limbs shunts cold and acidotic blood to the body's core, resulting in a drop of core temperature.

20. When the body is warmed and vasodilatation occurs, the depleted intravascular volume (secondary to cold diuresis) is insufficient. Hypoperfusion and shock (rewarming shock) then occurs.

Fill in the Blank

21. wind chill index

22. thermogenesis

23. cold diuresis

24. J

25. after drop phenomenon

Chapter 14
Case Study
Chief Concern

1. *What are some of the possible altitude sickness syndromes that would be suspected based on the mechanism of injury?*

   Any altitude above 12,000 feet is considered high altitude. Jay is at risk for acute mountain sickness including high altitude cerebral edema (HACE) and high altitude pulmonary edema (HAPE).

2. *How does Jay's origin impact the chances of his contracting altitude sickness?*

   Jay is starting from essentially sea level and rapidly going to high altitude. Without acclimatization to the altitude, Jay is at higher risk of developing one of these mountain sicknesses.

History

1. *What are the important elements of the history that a Paramedic should obtain?*

   After the chief concern, the Paramedic should use the standard SAMPLE history to determine if there is also dizziness, headache, nausea, fatigue, insomnia, or anorexia. Although some dyspnea on exertion is to be expected, more extreme dyspnea, especially at rest, bears further investigation.

2. *What questions should the Paramedic focus on in the medication history?*

   The Paramedic should inquire about the patient's use of alcohol, sleep medicine, and narcotics for pain management, as the medications in this trio all produce respiratory depression.

Examination

1. *What are the elements of the physical examination of a patient with suspected mountain sickness?*

   Following the primary assessment, the Paramedic should perform a complete cardiopulmonary examination. The Paramedic should focus on problems of respirations (i.e., hypoxia) as well as the cardiovascular compensation.

2. *Why is a neurological examination a critical element in this examination?*

   Suspected high altitude pulmonary edema can be accompanied by high altitude cerebral edema. Any signs of altered mental status (such as confusion) or signs resembling a stroke (like aphasia) may indicate high altitude cerebral edema.

Assessment

1. *What diagnosis did the Paramedic announce to the patient?*

   Based on the Lake Louise criteria, Jay had over half of the eight criterions for a diagnosis of high altitude pulmonary edema.

2. *What other diagnosis is commonly associated with this diagnosis?*

   High altitude cerebral edema is associated with high altitude pulmonary edema, although both can occur independently.

Treatment

1. *What is the first priority for patients with suspected mountain sickness?*

   The first treatment priority is descent. Getting the patient down 2,000 to 3,000 feet lower than the patient's current position is the goal.

2. *What are the priorities that follow?*

   Following descent, the Paramedic should administer oxygen as well as carefully monitor the patient's vital signs.

Evaluation

1. *What are some treatments for advanced HAPE?*

   Medications such as dexamethasone and nifedipine can be used to treat HAPE. These drugs can help to reduce pulmonary hypertension, which makes it difficult for the heart to pump.

2. *What is an experimental treatment that has shown promise in the treatment of advanced HAPE?*

   The use of the Gamow bag, a portable hyperbaric chamber, has shown promise in the treatment of advanced HAPE.

Disposition

1. *What is the most appropriate transport decision that will get the patient to definitive care?*

   The appropriate decision is to fly the patient to a facility that is familiar with treating mountain sickness, rather than transporting him to a local hospital.

2. *What are some of the transportation considerations?*

   Helicopter evacuation is often in order, in part due to the wilderness nature of the emergency. However, helicopters often have limited operational capacity, in which case the patient must be brought down to the helicopter's maximum ceiling.

Practice Questions
Multiple Choice

1. b
2. a
3. a
4. a
5. b
6. b
7. c
8. d
9. b
10. c
11. b
12. a
13. b
14. a
15. a

Short Answer

16. In acclimatization, the climber spends time at various altitudes to allow his body to adjust to the pressure changes. Over time, the body compensates for the reduction in oxygen by increasing red blood cells (polycythemia).

17. The three compensations for altitude-induced hypoxia are hyperventilation, polycythemia, and increased 2,3-DPG levels on the hemoglobin.

18. Cheyne–Stokes breathing is the result of the two respiratory drives—hypercapnia and hypoxia—competing with each other.

19. To differentiate a headache from dehydration from a headache from HACE, the patient should drink a liter of water and take a NSAID. If the headache resolves, it is probably due to dehydration.

20. Lack of oxygen causes high altitude retinal hemorrhage.

Fill in the Blank

21. Khumbu cough

22. snow blindness

23. Diamox

24. 2,3-DPG

25. acclimatization

Chapter 15

Case Study

Chief Concern

1. *What are some of the possible causes of sudden unconsciousness while underwater?*

   If the patient is unconscious and does not have a pulse, the assumption is that Andre experienced sudden cardiac death. If he is unconscious, but with a pulse, there are many possibilities, although the top of the list would have to be seizures or stroke.

2. *What is the implication of an emergency ascent?*

   An emergency ascent implicates a failure to properly decompress and therefore may lead to all of the associated decompression sicknesses, including DCS I and II.

History

1. *What are the important elements of the history that a Paramedic should obtain?*

   First, the Paramedic must assess the scene (i.e., fresh water versus salt, shallow diving versus deep diving). Another key question is water temperature and water contamination, especially if aspiration is a potential complication.

   A history of the present illness is necessary. For example, the Paramedic may determine if a convulsion was witnessed or if the patient suddenly became lax, suggesting a stroke. The Paramedic should also ascertain the dive depth, the submersion time, and the ascent time, if possible.

2. *What specific questions should the Paramedic ask, referring to the mechanism of injury?*

   There are risks associated with an emergency ascent, including pulmonary barotrauma. The Paramedic should ask if the patient has a history of COPD, spontaneous pneumothorax associated with blebs, history of pulmonary cysts, or tumors secondary to lung cancer. Patients with these conditions are prone to barotrauma and pneumothorax.

Examination

1. *What are the elements of the physical examination of a patient with suspected decompression sickness?*

   Beyond the essential primary assessment, the Paramedic should perform a neurological examination to assess for the most serious decompression illness, cerebral arterial gas embolism, as well as a cardiopulmonary examination to assess for barotrauma.

2. *Why is a 12-lead ECG a critical element in this examination?*

   Cold-water immersion has been known to cause dysrhythmia, particularly if the patient has a history of congenital prolonged QT syndrome. Therefore, it is essential for the Paramedic to do ECG monitoring and record a 12-lead ECG as a baseline.

Assessment

1. *What diagnosis did the Paramedic announce to the crew?*

   The symptom pattern is consistent with cerebral arterial gas embolism, but is also consistent with a stroke.

2. *What syndrome is suggested by the vital signs?*

   The vital signs suggest Cushing's triad and transtentorial herniation syndrome.

Treatment

1. *What is the national standard of care of patients with suspected decompression sickness, specifically cerebral arterial gas embolism?*

   In this case, the Paramedic is hard pressed to differentiate a stroke from CAGE. Fortunately, the care of both problems is the same: maintain an airway, provide ventilatory support as needed, or provide high-flow, high-concentration oxygen.

2. *What can be done if venous access is not readily obtainable?*

   Venous access should be obtained as soon as practical in case the patient seizes. In the interim, intranasal midazolam can be used to control seizure activity.

Evaluation

1. *What are some of the predictable complications associated with an emergency ascent?*

   Beyond the decompression sickness, there is also a risk of pulmonary barotrauma, such as a pneumothorax. Assisted ventilations may aggravate a pre-existing barotrauma. Aspiration of cold water can also lead to bronchorrhea and bronchospasm. This bronchospasm, in turn, can lead to further air trapping and pneumothorax.

2. *What are some of the concerns for a drowned diver?*

   Divers often dive in cold water (i.e., water that is not thermoneutral); therefore, they are at additional risk of hypothermia. The Paramedic should consider passive external rewarming after the removal of the patient's wet garments.

Disposition

1. *What is the most appropriate transport decision that will get the patient to definitive care?*

   Although the advantages of hyperbaric oxygen (HBO) seem obvious with suspected decompression sickness, this case is complicated by the question of stroke. Which occurred first: stroke, then rapid ascent, or unconsciousness, rapid ascent, and CAGE? The Paramedic should seek medical advice. If none is available, then the patient should be transported to the closest appropriate facility for stabilization.

2. *What is the optimal transportation decision?*

   The optimal transportation decision is to transport the patient to a stroke center with a hyperbaric chamber.

Practice Questions
Multiple Choice

1. d
2. d
3. a
4. b
5. c
6. d
7. a
8. a
9. d
10. d
11. a
12. b
13. c
14. a
15. c

Short Answer

16. If a person is murdered, the body does not aspirate before dying as occurs in a drowning. Therefore, the lungs remain full of air. As a result, the body remains positively buoyant and floats.

17. The difficulty with a patent foramen ovale arises when a diver ascends and nitrogen bubbles form in the venous circulation. Normally, these nitrogen bubbles are "filtered" out in the lungs. However, in the case of the patient with patent foramen ovale, the venous bubbles bypass the lungs, by moving from the right side of the heart to the left side of the heart through the patent foramen ovale, and on to the body and the brain. This leads to neurological symptoms such as weakness and dizziness.

18. The U.S. Navy has arbitrarily divided decompression sickness into two categories, though there is symptom crossover in both. The first category, decompression sickness I (DCS I), involves the skin and musculoskeletal system. DCS II includes neurological involvement and thus has more ominous implications.

19. The symptom pattern for decompression sickness is the bends, the staggers, the tingles, and the chokes.

20. During a too rapid, panic ascent, cerebral arterial gas embolism occurs, creating an embolic stroke.

Fill in the Blank

21. shallow water blackout
22. nitrogen narcosis
23. chokes
24. scotoma
25. cutis marmorata

Chapter 16
Case Study
Chief Concern

1. *What are some of the possible venomous marine life forms that a swimmer could encounter?*

   Venomous marine life is included in the phylum Cnidaria. There are four classes within the phylum, each with members that can potentially be toxic to humans. They are Hydrozoa (Portuguese man-o-war, fire coral), Cubozoa (box jellyfish), Anthozoa (sea anemone), and Scyphozoa (true jellyfish).

2. *Which of these marine life forms is not a jellyfish?*

   The Anthozoa, or sea anemone, is not a jellyfish.

History

1. *What are the important elements of the history that a Paramedic should obtain?*

   Following scene safety, the Paramedic should use the standard SAMPLE tool for history-gathering as well as identify the specifics of the incident (i.e., who, what, where, when, and how).

2. *What is the symptom pattern associated with a Portuguese man-o-war jellyfish bite?*

   The primary clinical effect is pain; however, the bite can also cause generalized weakness, limb numbness and tingling, nasal and ocular discharge, and muscle spasm.

Examination

1. *What are the elements of the physical examination of a patient with a suspected jellyfish sting?*

   Following the primary assessment and vital signs, the Paramedic should perform an complete examination of the patient's lower extremities, looking for sting markers. Vesicles and bullae can be present, with potential for skin necrosis in the affected areas.

2. *What other reactions might occur as a result of the envenomation?*

   In some cases, the patient may experience an anaphylactoid reaction and urticaria may be visible on the upper chest.

Assessment

1. *What diagnosis did the Paramedic announce to the patient?*

   Based on local information, the patient's description of the event, and the physical examination findings, the sting is probably from a Portuguese man-o-war. The Paramedic's diagnosis would be marine life envenomation, most likely from a Portuguese man-o-war.

2. *What secondary diagnosis might be associated with the primary diagnosis?*

   A secondary diagnosis may be a possible anaphylactoid reaction to the venom.

Treatment

1. *What is the national standard of care of patients with suspected marine envenomation?*

   Treatment should first be directed at preventing further firing of nematocysts. Vinegar or acetic acid (4% to 6%) is a commonly accepted treatment to prevent further nematocyst discharge. The vinegar should be poured over the affected area with adherent tentacles for at least 30 seconds. After treatment with vinegar, the Paramedic can remove the tentacles.

2. *What are some of the patient-specific concerns and considerations that the Paramedic should consider when applying this plan of care for patients presenting with suspected marine envenomation?*

   The prehospital treatment of Cnidarian bites initially involves decreasing the risk of further injury to the patient or rescuer. If entering the water to rescue an individual, the rescuer should wear protective clothing to keep from being envenomed. Furthermore, the rescuer should only attempt a rescue if trained in water rescue.

Evaluation

1. *What are some of the predictable complications associated with a sting from the Portuguese man-o-war?*

   Nematocysts can remain active for hours and can continue pain even without physical contact with the man-o-war.

2. *What is the treatment to prevent these complications?*

   The nematocysts from the Portuguese man-o-war can be inactivated by hot water (100°F to 113°F). If unable to measure the water temperature, the Paramedic should use the hottest water the patient can tolerate. Hot water immersion, or rinsing in the shower, should continue for 20 minutes.

Disposition

1. *What is the most appropriate transport decision that will get the patient to definitive care?*

   Patients with suspected envenomation should be transported to the closest appropriate facility.

2. *What if the patient refuses further care or transport?*

   Because symptoms from envenomations can be delayed, it is important to encourage patients to go to the hospital, even if they are feeling well.

Practice Questions
Multiple Choice

1. d
2. d
3. a
4. b
5. b
6. a
7. b
8. d
9. a
10. a
11. c
12. b
13. a
14. d
15. a

Short Answer

16. Alpha-latrotoxin injected by the black widow spider is a neurotoxin that causes opening of presynaptic cation channels, causing release of neurotransmitters, specifically calcium. The large amount of neurotransmitters causes significant stimulation at the motor endplate of the neuromuscular junction with resultant physical findings.

17. Scorpion toxins are active on the voltage-gated ion channels at the neuromuscular junction, and primarily affect sodium channels. This causes the repetitive firing of both sympathetic and parasympathetic nerves, allowing for release of acetylcholine and catecholamines.

18. Tourniquets should be avoided when treating snake bites as they can cause significant tissue ischemia and necrosis.

19. Treatment should first be directed at preventing further firing of nematocysts. Vinegar or acetic acid (4% to 6%) is a commonly accepted treatment to prevent further nematocyst discharge. The Paramedic should pour the vinegar over the affected area with adherent tentacles for at least 30 seconds. After treatment with vinegar, the Paramedic can remove the tentacles.

20. Seabather's eruption is a cutanous, pruritic reaction to the larvae of the thimble jellyfish, *Linuche unguiculata*. The eruption typically occurs underneath the bathing suit, which is believed to trap the jellyfish larvae against the skin.

Fill in the Blank

21. hemolysin
22. triangular
23. coral
24. latrodectus facies
25. necrotic arachnidism

Chapter 17

Case Study

1. *What are the vehicle safety standards for ambulance construction?*

   The only nationally approved safety standard that is applicable to ambulances is the American National Standards Institute and American Society of Safety Engineers standard Z15.1 fleet safety standard.

2. *What can be done to make the patient compartment safer for all of the occupants?*

   The patient compartment can be made safer by securing loose equipment (particularly oxygen bottles and ECG monitors), providing forward-facing seats that have laps belts for EMS providers, and softening head strike surfaces with shock-absorbing materials.

3. *What safety performance modifications to an ambulance will increase its crashworthiness?*

   Among the modifications that may improve safety is development of a crashworthy patient compartment complete with crumple zones, as well as intelligent transportation systems that can modify potentially dangerous driving behaviors, such as is possible with in-vehicle telematics technology.

4. *What liability does the service hold if this ambulance is involved in a crash? What is the likelihood that they will be sued?*

   Failure to institute policies and procedures (based on research findings) that may improve EMS provider survival in the event of an ambulance collision can leave companies, both volunteer and proprietary, and municipalities open to charges of negligence. Current trends in EMS litigation have put equipment failure, including ambulance construction, at the top of the list of potential suits.

Practice Questions

Multiple Choice

1. a
2. a
3. d
4. d
5. b
6. b
7. c
8. a
9. a
10. a
11. a
12. d
13. d
14. c
15. d

Short Answer

16. When designing head protection for EMS, designers need to consider the Paramedic's communications capability with both patients and the driver; stethoscope auscultation; its effectiveness in high horizontal G forces, such as an automotive crash;, the ability for others to identify the responder; and functional options such as making it lightweight and low profile, providing biohazard protection, allowing adequate visibility, and providing an internal visor to enhance image enhancing.

17. The color for peak night sensitivity is blue-green, whereas the color for peak day sensitivity is yellow-green.

18. The National Institute for Occupational Safety and Health (NIOSH) is an organization that is historically geared toward epidemiology, biohazards, and ergonomic research.

19. When wearing dark blue uniforms at night, EMS providers can be "camouflaged" by the vehicle's pattern, particularly the Battenberg vehicle pattern, or not seen at all.

20. In-vehicle telematics technology provides drivers with real time monitoring and feedback of their driving performance.

Fill in the Blank

21. Federal Motor Vehicle Safety

22. Battenberg

23. helmet

24. Worker Visibility

25. KKK

Chapter 18
Case Study

1. *What are some of the possible advantages of helicopter transport?*

   The advantages of air medical transport by helicopter are twofold: the time saved by faster flight and the higher quality of care that can be brought to the field.

2. *What conditions warrant air medical service?*

   The list of conditions is long and detailed. The National Association of EMS Physicians lists the criteria in their position paper; it includes significant trauma such as falling from a great height.

3. *What is the most appropriate transport decision that will get the patient to definitive care?*

   Owing to the time-sensitive nature of serious trauma (i.e., the golden hour), the most appropriate decision is air medical transport.

4. *What are the advantages of transporting a patient with suspected trauma to these hospitals, even if that means bypassing other hospitals in the process?*

   Studies have shown that transportation to a trauma center markedly improves patient survival, sometimes by as much as 50%.

Practice Questions
Multiple Choice

1. c
2. c
3. a
4. a
5. b
6. d
7. a
8. d
9. d
10. b
11. b
12. d
13. c
14. d
15. d

Short Answer

16. Cones, flares, headlights, and other secured markers can be used to mark a landing zone. Strobe lights should not be used.

17. The height of the helicopter's main rotor blades may require that approaching personnel duck down to avoid being struck by them. For this reason, it is a good practice for a Paramedic to wear a safety helmet whenever he is around an aircraft.

18. If the pilot signals the Paramedic to approach the aircraft, he should always approach from the front (the 12 o'clock position), within clear view of the pilot. Personnel should never approach a helicopter from the rear (the 6 o'clock position).

19. The Centers for Disease Control (CDC) has defined a culture of safety as the shared commitment of management and employees to ensure the safety of the work environment.

20. The Commission for Accreditation of Medical Transport Services (CAMTS) has self-imposed requirements reflected in their standards. These are considered by many to be the national standard for practice in the air medical industry.

Fill in the Blank

21. auto-launch

22. rotor wash

23. wave-off

24. hot load

25. rotor wing

Chapter 19
Case Study

1. *What are some of the possible complications that the Paramedic may encounter en route to the receiving hospital?*

   This boy is at great risk for hemorrhagic shock secondary to the injuries that he sustained. Furthermore, the patient has pulmonary complications (i.e., pneumothorax) that can deteriorate into a tension pneumothorax.

2. *What is the "problem list" that the Paramedic must monitor?*

   The Paramedic must monitor the patient's hemodynamic status carefully. The use of an arterial line would be very helpful. The Paramedic must also monitor the patient's pneumothorax, as well as the chest tube assembly.

3. *What is the most appropriate transport decision that will get the patient to definitive care?*

   This patient is critically ill and will need the services of a pediatric intensive care unit if he is going to survive. The first choice for transportation is likely air medical. In some cases, air medical is not available (i.e., weather conditions, other missions, etc.). In that case, ground transport via ambulance is in order.

4. *What are the advantages of transporting a patient with suspected spinal cord injury to these hospitals, even if that means bypassing other hospitals in the process?*

   Regional trauma centers have been shown to decrease morbidity and mortality in this special population. The pediatric population represents a subset of the larger population that has even more special needs and the need for specialized equipment that may only be available in a pediatric trauma center.

Practice Questions
Multiple Choice

1. d
2. a
3. c
4. a
5. c
6. c
7. d
8. c
9. b
10. c
11. a
12. b
13. c
14. a
15. a

Short Answer

16. Specialization of hospitals refers to the concept of special hospital designations for trauma, which allows the resources for managing critically injured patients to be concentrated at strategically located centers in a given region.

17. Reverse dumping is a hospital's refusal of patients for transfer from another facility. Dumping, a hospital's refusal of original admission due to an inability to pay, was reversed by EMTALA.

18. EMTALA defines "stabilized" as a physical state in which a patient will not likely deteriorate during transfer.

19. A specialty care transport Paramedic has training above the level of a typical Paramedic.

20. Protocols are intended for patients with a symptom complex that suggests either a disorder or a syndrome that leads to a rudimentary field diagnosis, whereas patient care guidelines are the instructions for the intended continuance of care for patients with an established medical diagnosis.

Fill in the Blank

21. specialty care transport

22. hemolytic reaction

23. Emergency Medical Treatment Active Labor Act

24. patient care guidelines

25. phlebostatic axis

Chapter 20

Case Study

1. *What is the National Response Framework for a mass-casualty incident?*

   The National Response Plan contains 15 Emergency Support Functions designed to be called up for any disaster. These 15 scenarios were anticipated in the National Preparedness Guidelines.

2. *What law empowers the federal government to activate reservists and disaster teams, as well as call for volunteers?*

   The three pivotal laws are the Stafford Act of 1974, the Homeland Security Act of 2002, and the Post-Katrina Emergency Management Reform Act of 2007.

3. *What is the Strategic National Stockpile?*

   The Strategic National Stockpile contains materials, such as the CHEMPACK, that may be needed in the event of a disaster. EMS CHEMPACKs are capable of treating 400 casualties.

4. *What is the Medical Reserve Corps?*

   The Medical Reserve Corps (MRC) program is a volunteer program for medical professionals administered by the Department of Health and Human Services. The MRC organizes public health, medical, and other volunteers who want to donate their time and expertise to prepare for and respond to emergencies. Volunteer MRC units accomplish this mission by supplementing existing emergency and public health resources during a disaster.

Practice Questions
Multiple Choice

1. d
2. a
3. c
4. d

5. d
6. d
7. a
8. a

9. a

10. a

11. a

12. d

13. d

14. d

15. a

Short Answer

16. The Posse Comitatus Act (18 U.S.C.) prevents the Army or Air Force from being used in a law enforcement capacity within the United States.

17. Specialty disaster response teams are the Veterinary Medical Assistance Team, the National Pharmacy Response Team, the Disaster Mortuary Operational Response Team, and the National Nurse Response Team.

18. The Strategic National Stockpile (SNS) is designed to supplement and re-supply state and local public health agencies in the event of a national emergency. The Strategic National Stockpile contains antibiotics, chemical antidotes, antitoxins, life-support medications, IV and airway maintenance supplies, and other medical/surgical items.

19. CHEMPACK is a component of the Strategic National Stockpile. The CHEMPACK program establishes caches of nerve agent and other antidotes in selected cities.

20. The federal government sponsors Community Emergency Response Teams (CERT) to augment emergency responders following a disaster. CERTs prepare people to help themselves, their families, and their neighbors in the event of a disaster in their community. Community Emergency Response Team volunteers learn about disaster preparedness and basic disaster response, such as fire safety, light search and rescue, and disaster medical operations.

Fill in the Blank

21. National Response Plan

22. Joint Information Center

23. Mobile Emergency Response Support

24. Urban Search and Rescue

25. Disaster Medical Assistance Team

Chapter 21

Case Study

1. *What is the implication of multiple patients with the same symptoms?*

   Multiple patients with the same or similar symptom pattern may indicate a cluster. These clusters can occur around dispersal points for biological weapons.

2. *What protection should the Paramedic take against these forms of terrorism?*

   Using the concepts of distance, shielding, and time, the Paramedic should use standard infectious disease precautions including the use of personal protective equipment (i.e., shielding).

3. *What is the preferred response to a terrorist threat?*

   Remaining vigilant, the Paramedic should identify perceived clusters to the proper authorities. In many instances, hospitals have established reporting mechanisms that can identify a cluster. However, in cities with multiple hospitals, the commonality that is involved in multiple casualties may be EMS.

4. *Why would terrorists use an infectious agent as the weapon of choice?*

Terrorists may use biological agents because they are difficult to detect, allowing the terrorists to flee; they are difficult to contain, promoting panic in the public; and they strike at a critical infrastructure that is already strained (i.e., health care and hospitals).

Practice Questions
Multiple Choice

1. a
2. c
3. d
4. b
5. a
6. d
7. c
8. d

9. a
10. c
11. a
12. d
13. b
14. a
15. d

Short Answer

16. A philosophical definition of terrorism by C. A. J. Coady is "the tactic of intentionally targeting non-combatants . . . with lethal or severe violence . . . meant to produce political results via the creation of fear."

17. The right-wing cherishes individual freedoms over government regulations, often declaring a racist and radical supremacy while embracing antigovernment and antiregulatory platforms. Two of the most currently active right-wing groups are the anti-abortionists and the self-proclaimed militia.

18. The left-wing extremists are traditionally anticapitalists, with some having an anarchist philosophy that rejects the idea of private property and organized government.

19. The mnemonic used for organophosphate poisoning is SLUDGEM or DUMBELS.

20. Blood agents are cellular asphyxiants that inhibit the body's ability to exchange gasses.

Fill in the Blank

21. situational awareness
22. cluster
23. dirty bomb

24. pralidoxime chloride
25. secondary devices

Chapter 22
Case Study

1. *How does triage differ in a public health emergency?*

Triage in a public health emergency is likely to occur in several locations and may focus on exposure and prophylaxis rather than treatment. Furthermore, triage during a public health emergency tends to escalate as time progresses to a nadir that may be days or even weeks later.

2. *What are some techniques used to prevent the spread of an infectious disease?*

The key to preventing the spread of disease is to separate the infected population from the noninfected population. This can be accomplished by isolation and/or social distancing.

3. *What "out of scope of practice" duties might a Paramedic perform in this situation?*

Paramedics may be requested to either perform atypical skills, such as public vaccinations, or perform routine skills in an unusual place, such as a hospital.

4. *What training could Paramedics perform that would prepare them for these roles?*

To prepare for public vaccinations, Paramedics may participate in routine flu season immunizations at local clinics. This simulates point of dispersal (POD) activity. Alternatively, Paramedics may participate in live drills of public health emergencies such as community triage exercises.

Practice Questions
Multiple Choice

1. c	9. d
2. b	10. b
3. a	11. b
4. c	12. a
5. c	13. c
6. a	14. d
7. c	15. b
8. d	

Short Answer

16. The core ethical principle of public health is, "The needs of the many may outweigh the needs to the few."

17. A public health emergency is a poorly demarcated, potentially escalating event that impacts the health and well-being of the citizens.

18. The challenges to public health during an emergency are inadequate funding, inadequate personnel, scarcity of medical supplies, communications difficulties, and public panic.

19. An all-hazards approach assumes commonality in all public health emergencies and utilizes a general response plan that is modified for specific situations as they arise.

20. Examples of training for a public health emergency include classroom training, tabletop exercises, on-line exercises, and live drills.

Fill in the Blank

21. index case	24. social distancing
22. point of dispensing	25. ring vaccination
23. isolation	

Chapter 23

Case Study

1. *What is the first type of triage that the Paramedics would use?*

   The Paramedics would perform an extrication triage.

2. *What are the disadvantages of this first triage?*

   The extrication triage is done without full knowledge of the conditions of all of the patients. The level of triage assigned will be altered as more is known about the numbers and conditions of patients as well as the available resources.

3. *What are some complications of inappropriate triage?*

   Underestimating the severity of a patient's wounds can result in undertriage and increased morbidity and mortality. Alternatively, overestimation of the severity of a patient's wounds can result in overtriage and increased morbidity and mortality.

4. *Name a problem associated with the START triage.*

   The START triage system includes the patient's ability to walk. If a patient cannot walk (e.g., due to a broken leg) but is otherwise stable (i.e., normal respirations, pulse, and mentation), the patient may be incorrectly "upgraded."

Practice Questions

Multiple Choice

1. a
2. b
3. a
4. d
5. b
6. c
7. b
8. c
9. b
10. a
11. d
12. d
13. c
14. a
15. d

Short Answer

16. The goal of triage is to get the most patients to the most appropriate care.

17. The shift from the worst first to the greatest good for the greatest number occurred in World War I with the advent of weapons of mass destruction.

18. SALT is the Sort–Assess–Lifesaving interventions–Treat/transport triage system created by the federal Centers for Disease Control. It is a two-step process of sorting and treating.

19. The Sacco system (STM) uses evidence-based methodology, based on 76,000 patients in a trauma registry, for its triage scheme.

20. Triage is performed at multiple junctures in the emergency response system. One tool used is the Secondary Assessment of Victim Endpoint (SAVE).

Fill in the Blank

21. worst first
22. undertriage
23. overtriage
24. expectant
25. jumpSTART

Chapter 24

Case Study

1. *What are the Paramedic's first responsibilities on the scene of a motor vehicle collision?*

   The Paramedic's first responsibility on the scene of any motor vehicle collision is to ensure personal safety by donning personal protective equipment, such as ANSI-rated safety vests.

2. *What are the initial actions the Paramedic should take to immobilize the vehicle?*

   The vehicle can be immobilized by putting chocks in front of and behind the tires, placing the vehicle in park, or engaging the emergency brake.

3. *What are some typical "space-making" techniques that a Paramedic can implement prior to the arrival of heavy rescue?*

   Space-making techniques include tilting the steering wheel, sliding the chair backwards, rolling the window down, and even reclining the seat.

4. *What are the implications of new hybrid drivetrains?*

   Hybrid drivetrains use a conventional gas engine to power either batteries or an electric engine. These high-voltage electrical systems carry high voltage, are colored orange, and should never be cut.

Practice Questions

Multiple Choice

1. b
2. c
3. a
4. b
5. b
6. a
7. d
8. a
9. c
10. b
11. d
12. b
13. a
14. d
15. c

Short Answer

16. Disentanglement is the act of cutting the vehicle away from the patient, whereas extrication is the act of removing the patient from the vehicle.

17. ROPS is rollover protection, generally provided through steel-reinforced cages placed over the driver and passengers.

18. In a modified dash roll, the dash is rolled forward using a short ram or spreaders. Several strategic cuts must be made in the dash before the dash is rolled.

19. One of the most effective methods of maximizing interior space is the cross-ramming evolution, in which the hydraulic ram is placed into the vehicle and then extended from one vehicle component to another.

20. Hybrid drivetrains combine a gasoline or diesel engine with an electric motor.

Fill in the Blank

21. protective envelope
22. 15
23. fuel cells
24. supplemental restraint systems
25. pretensioners

Chapter 25

Case Study

1. *What are the two philosophical components of the rehabilitation standard?*

   The first philosophical component of the rehabilitation standard is that firefighters have insight into their own need for hydration, rest, and nutrition. The second philosophical component is that incident commanders must delegate authority to Paramedics to keep firefighters from returning to service if, in their professional judgment, the firefighter is not fit to return to duty.

2. *What organizations are covered under the rehabilitation standard?*

   The rehabilitation standard applies to rescue teams, fire suppression teams, emergency medical services, hazardous materials teams, special operations, and industrial fire brigades.

3. *What actions will provide "relief from climatic conditions"?*

   Relief from climatic conditions involves routing responders to a separate area, building, or tent that gets them out of the wind, smoke, dust, and direct sunlight, thereby permitting them to get some privacy and rest.

4. *What is the most effective active cooling system?*

   Although misting tents, forearm immersion chairs, and cooling vests are effective, the most effective and cost-effective system may be the cold towel method, which involves placing cold towels around the patient's head and/or neck.

Practice Questions

Multiple Choice

1. a
2. c
3. b
4. b
5. b
6. b
7. c
8. b
9. b
10. b
11. c
12. d
13. d
14. d
15. d

Short Answer

16. The NFPA 1584 standards in the 2008 version are based on the premise that firefighters need to make their own decisions about hydration, rest, and nutrition.

17. Rehabilitation is any action to bring a person back to her near normal physiological condition. It is required in any situation where a reasonable risk to safety and/or health exists for any responder.

18. The supplies needed for a cold towel cooling system in rehabilitation are ice, water, bleach, towels, and plastic buckets. Five gallon buckets that can be obtained from a local hardware or home improvement store work best for this operation. Initially, the Paramedic fills a bucket with water and adds ice until a comfortable temperature is achieved. If ice is not immediately available, cool water can be used alone. The Paramedic places dry towels into the water-filled bucket. Once wet, they should be wrung out until damp (not dripping).

19. Medical monitoring refers to observation of firefighter team members for adverse health effects of firefighting including heat or cold stress, physical and psychological stress, and environmental stress.

20. NFPA 1584 specifies that members entering and leaving rehabilitation will be accounted for through the personnel accountability system being used by the incident commander in charge of the scene.

Fill in the Blank

21. incident commander

22. wind chill, heat stress

23. water

24. three

25. medical monitoring

Chapter 26
Case Study

1. *What will help the first responder identify the contents of the building?*

   Buildings containing potentially hazardous materials should display the NFPA standard 704 placard on the building. This placard identifies the reactivity, flammability, and health hazards of the most dangerous chemical as well as special instructions such as "don't add water."

2. *Why would knowing the vapor density of the burning material be important?*

   Knowing the vapor density helps the Paramedic predict whether the chemical gasses are lighter than air or heavier than air.

3. *What information does the IDLH system provide?*

   The immediately dangerous to life and health (IDLH) system, created by the EPA and NIOSH, defines concentration levels that will cause unconsciousness, incapacitation, or adverse health effects.

4. *What are the advantages of on-scene decontamination?*

   Many hospitals have limited or no capacity to perform decontamination on-scene. Bringing a contaminated patient to the emergency department may potentially spread contamination to other patients.

Practice Questions
Multiple Choice

1. a

2. c

3. d

4. b

5. a

6. c

7. a

8. c

9. d

10. b

11. d

12. c

13. b

14. a

15. c

Short Answer

16. Hazardous materials are defined as any substance (solid, liquid, or gas) that, when released, is capable of creating harm to people, the environment, or property.

17. Compressed gas is a vapor with an absolute pressure of greater than 40 pounds per square inch (psi).

18. Vapor density is the concentration of a gas when compared to air.

19. The threshold limit values—short-term exposure limit is the maximum acceptable exposure a person can endure without apparent ill effects after 15 minutes of exposure.

20. A medical surveillance plan typically has three elements: baseline, exposure specific, and on-scene rehabilitation.

Fill in the Blank

21. *Emergency Response Guide*

22. flash point

23. lower explosive limit

24. higher explosive limit

25. pyrophorics

Chapter 27

Case Study

1. *Under what authority does federal Urban Search and Rescue operate?*

   Urban Search and Rescue (USAR) is a part of the Federal Response Plan and is the responsibility of the Department of Homeland Security.

2. *How many USAR teams are there?*

   There are 25 USAR teams with 70 people and four canines apiece, strategically located across the United States. These teams are referred to as task forces in the incident management system.

3. *How does the technical USAR team operate?*

   The structural engineers within a technical team evaluate the structure for active and potential collapse, work with hazardous materials specialists to identify hazards, and work with heavy equipment and rigging specialists to mitigate those hazards so rescuers can rescue patients.

4. *How does the medical USAR team operate?*

   The medical team is led by physicians, who serve as medical team managers, and care is performed by Paramedics, in the role of medical specialists. The medical team is trained to treat conditions likely to be encountered in the USAR environment, including crush injury. The medical team must also care for the canines in the unit as well as team members.

Practice Questions
Multiple Choice

1. a
2. a
3. c
4. c
5. b
6. c
7. a
8. c
9. d
10. a
11. d
12. d
13. c
14. d
15. c

Short Answer

16. Confined space is an enclosed area with limited access that is not designed for human occupancy. It has the potential to cause physical, chemical, or atmospheric injury.

17. Heavy construction is capable of withstanding horizontal forces and shear forces, whereas light construction is designed to only withstand vertical forces.

18. Rostered three deep means that there are three people to each station or post, to guarantee availability and facilitate rapid deployment.

19. With a rescue there is an expectation of patient survival, whereas with a recovery the person is presumed dead.

20. The technical team is comprised of the following specialists: hazardous materials, structural, and heavy equipment and rigging.

Fill in the Blank

21. I

22. rescue specialists

23. medical team managers, medical specialists

24. rescue, recovery

25. crush syndrome

Chapter 28

Case Study

1. *What are the types of water rescue?*

   Water rescue can occur in surface water, calm water, or swift water. Many water rescues occur in flood waters.

2. *What are the different types of water search methods?*

   There are two methods for water search. The first uses passive search measures, such as shore-based rescues using throw bags, Sheppard's crooks, and ring buoys. The other water search method uses either boat-based rescue or water entry. Both methods require special training.

3. *What are the dangers in swift water rescue?*

   The three dangers in swift water rescue are low-head dams, which create hydraulic currents; foot entrapments created by underwater debris; and entrapment in strainers in the river.

4. *What safety measures are taken during a swift water rescue?*

   Normally, several rope lines are extended across the water. One is a droop line, which is draped from a bridge to snag a passing patient. Another line is the ferry line or tension diagonal, which stretches across the water to snag a passing patient and draw him to the shore. Two-line taglines are also used for safety.

Practice Questions

Multiple Choice

1. a
2. a
3. a
4. b
5. a
6. b
7. c
8. c
9. d
10. a
11. a
12. c
13. d
14. c
15. d

Short Answer

16. Differential pressure is the force of two bodies of water at different elevations trying to equalize.

17. A person assumes the defensive swimming position by lying on the back, facing downstream.

18. The greatest danger to rescuers in fast water is foot entrapments, as they can frequently cause ankle fractures. Larger rocks create holes and crevices that rescuers may step into when they plant a foot to step. The loss of balance and the current force can pull the rescuer downstream while pinning the foot between the rocks.

19. The most common surf entrapment is getting into a rip current. Rip currents are formed when water being pushed inshore finds a place to drain back out. Since the rip current is draining water back out offshore, swimming against it is likened to running on a treadmill.

20. Triangulation is using different lines of sight to narrow down a location. It is very effective if the witnesses are interviewed from where they saw the events.

Fill in the Blank

21. low head, hydraulic current

22. surging waves

23. personal flotation device

24. heat escape lessening position

25. strainers

Chapter 29
Case Study

1. *What National Fire Protection Association standard relates to wilderness search and rescue?*

   The NFPA standard 1670 speaks to the need for the agency having jurisdiction over an area to plan and prepare for SAR. This includes assembling a set of operational procedures and making preparations, which may include gathering equipment and training responders.

2. *What are the levels of SAR responders?*

   The first level is the Awareness level, where the Paramedic is expected to recognize the need for wilderness search and rescue. The next level is the Operations level, where the Paramedic is expected to perform a scene size-up and execute the preplan. The last level is the Technician level, where the Paramedic is expected to be able to perform the searches including rope rescue as well as shore-based water rescue.

3. *What are the rudimentary searches performed at the beginning of the search and rescue operation?*

   The two rudimentary searches are the hasty search (a quick trail walk spent looking for clues) and the bastard search (a quick look at places that might be attractive to the lost person).

4. *What is tracking?*

   With a clue in hand, the lead person (pointer) proceeds to look for more signs (i.e., evidence the patient passed that way). Using flankers, the pointer can move quickly to determine the patient's speed and direction.

Practice Questions
Multiple Choice

1. c
2. a
3. c

4. d
5. c
6. d

7. a

8. a

9. c

10. b

11. b

12. a

13. c

14. d

15. d

Short Answer

16. A study of 2,302 wilderness search and rescue (SAR) missions conducted by Adams et al. and published in the *Journal of Wilderness and Environmental Medicine* in 2007 indicated that "time alone was the strongest predictor of survival."

17. A hasty search is a search of "high probability" areas first.

18. A bastard search involves looking for any place that can provide food, water, shelter, or medical attention.

19. Clue consciousness is high awareness of potential field clues and the mindset that clues can come from unexpected sources.

20. Sign cutting is the actual search for evidence that a subject has been in the area and establishing a point from which to track.

Fill in the Blank

21. probability of area

22. point last seen

23. sole signature

24. woods shock

25. searcher rehabilitation

Chapter 30
Case Study

1. *What is a hazard analysis?*

   As the definition of technical rescue suggests, any tower, multistory building, farm silo, cave, or sewer system has the potential to be the site for a technical rescue and should be included in the hazard analysis for the agency having jurisdiction.

2. *What is a slope analysis?*

   When reviewing the terrain—whether on foot, by map, or by Earth satellite photographs—the rescuer performs a slope analysis to determine the degree of hazard in the jurisdiction and the need for specialized rope rescue teams.

3. *What National Fire Protection Association standards relate to operations and training for technical rescue?*

   The NFPA 1670 standard involves operations and training for technical search and rescue incidents.

4. *What National Fire Protection Association standards relate to technical rescue equipment?*

   The NFPA standard 1983 speaks to harnesses, ropes, and even carabiners. The standards establish load limits, breaking strengths, and other safety requirements for the professional rescue operation.

Practice Questions

Multiple Choice

1. d
2. b
3. d
4. b
5. c
6. a
7. c
8. a
9. a
10. d
11. d
12. a
13. a
14. d
15. a

Short Answer

16. Only ropes that are designated as life safety ropes—that is, designed to support a life load during an emergency—should be used in rescue.

17. A belay is a second rope used to protect the rescuer from a fall. Originally, a belay meant to make fast (i.e., to secure a rope from moving). In this case, a belay is meant to make the rescuer secure.

18. Mechanical advantage is a simple machine that multiplies the force put into it. The formula is length of arm divided by length of resistance arm.

19. The most effective hauling system is the 3:1 Z rig. The rope forms a Z pattern as it winds between two pulleys that are pulled closer together. Thus, a moderately efficient pulley (friction always plays a role in efficiency) can make lifting 200 pounds feel like lifting 91 pounds. A 3:1 simple pulley system is so commonly used that many rescuers "preset" the system in a hauling system.

20. To prevent the patient from falling out of the basket, the rescuer must secure the patient to the basket. For low angle ascents, the patient may be "zippered" into the basket with webbing. Taking a long length of webbing secured by a hitch at one end, the two free ends of the webbing are weaved back and forth over the patient. However, in most cases, the patient is secured into the basket with a seat harness (often an improvised one) or a chest harness. These harnesses are especially important in high angle or vertical ascent. (Vertical ascent may be necessary in confined spaces.)

Fill in the Blank

21. highline
22. rigging plate
23. descent control device
24. load distributing anchor
25. sling

Chapter 31

Case Study

1. *What aspects should be considered in event preplanning?*

   There are three main aspects to consider in event preplanning: the biomedical, the psychosocial, and the environmental. The biomedical includes issues related to age and predictable medical emergencies. The psychosocial includes issues related to the crowd sentiment and the presence of alcohol and/or drugs on-scene. The environmental includes issues related to the physical layout of the property as well as weather.

2. *What is the role of public health?*

   Public health is concerned with food preparation, water safety, and waste management.

3. *What are examples of "early warning systems" for medical emergencies?*

   Early warning systems can range from expensive electronic surveillance with cameras to human spotters with binoculars. Roving teams have also been shown to be highly effective.

4. *What on-scene care should be available?*

   In some cases, a concession stand provided by the local pharmacy will take care of a large number of complaints (sunburn, blisters, and headache). A forward aid station can help to stabilize patients (i.e., a way station) or provide care for minor medical emergencies. A field hospital can serve as a collecting point for patients for off-site transportation or as a temporary holding area to mitigate surges of admissions at the hospitals.

Practice Questions
Multiple Choice

1. d
2. d
3. b
4. d
5. b
6. d
7. a
8. d

9. c
10. d
11. d
12. d
13. c
14. d
15. d

Short Answer

16. The goal of mass-gathering medicine is to mitigate the predictable perils and, when that is not possible, to provide timely emergency medical care.

17. TEAM is an educational program that teaches the skills necessary for a concessionaire, or a Paramedic, to identify an intoxicated individual and to intervene in a "nonconfrontational way" to ensure the safety of the attendee and the staff.

18. Human stampedes have been reported when large numbers of people in close proximity press together. Compressive forces from "penned in" participants can be greater than one-half ton as people pile on, either vertically or horizontally. Severe traumas and trauma arrests from compressive asphyxiation (known as crowd crush) are not uncommon during a human stampede.

19. Following a credible threat, the first step in mass evacuation is warning the public. The use of pre-existing public address systems is an option as well as the use of the media. It may be possible at entertainment events to use the sound system. In those instances where public address systems are not available, telecommunicators will need to use existing resources to notify the public, such as the public address feature of the siren of an ambulance or patrol car. Carefully prepared scripts can be given to strategically placed units that control the movement of the crowd and help to prevent crowd surge.

20. The event profile contains information about the type of event, such as whether it is indoors or outdoors, and whether it is restricted (such as fenced in) or extended (with a capability of expanding beyond the grounds). Crowd information should also be provided, such as whether the crowd will be seated or mobile and the anticipated sentiment of the crowd (passive, active, or energetic). The teams should also be provided with expectations of crowd size. Published information about the duration of the event and the times for special events (e.g., when a headliner is expected to perform at a rock concert) should be provided. Policies regarding alcohol consumption should also be furnished in the event profile brief.

    Finally, the extended forecast for the day of the event, which includes the expected high temperature and humidity, should be included along with a map of the grounds. This map should have the location of crowd barriers, pathways, and exits clearly marked. Access points to bounded areas should also be marked.

Fill in the Blank

21. 1,000

22. crowd sentiment

23. patient load

24. compressive asphyxiation

25. mass evacuation

Chapter 32
Case Study

1. *What are the four missions of the tactical medic?*

   The missions of the tactical medic are preventative medical care for law enforcement officers, medical threat assessment prior to operations, emergency medical support during operations, and medical direction/oversight of law enforcement special operations.

2. *What are the advantages of hospital-based medical support? EMS/Fire-based medical support? Law enforcement-based medical support?*

   Hospital-based tactical medical support has the benefit of on-site physicians providing medical control, although they are unfamiliar with prehospital operations. EMS/Fire-based operations have the advantage of knowledge of prehospital care and packaging, although they are unfamiliar with police routines. Law enforcement-based operations are familiar with police traditions, habits, and routines, but are not familiar with prehospital care and transportation.

3. *If EMS is not medically trained, then under what conditions must they operate at the scene of a tactical operation?*

   Untrained Paramedics operate in the cool zone, a relatively safe zone free of direct fire where staging occurs. The Paramedics must be afforded both cover (i.e., protection from projectiles) as well as concealment.

4. *What is the minimum equipment needed for a Paramedic to operate in the cool zone?*

   Technically, the Paramedic can operate in the cool zone with standard EMS equipment. However, the volatile nature of tactical operations, and subsequent shifting of zones, makes it prudent to provide the Paramedic with at least a ballistic helmet and vest.

Practice Questions
Multiple Choice

1. b

2. a

3. d

4. a

5. a

6. c

7. a

8. c

9. a

10. c

11. a

12. c

13. a

14. c

15. d

Short Answer

16. Tactical EMS is medical support for tactical law enforcement operations.

17. Sustained medical operations can be broken up into two broad categories. Short-term missions are those lasting approximately one week, whereas long-term missions refer to anything lasting longer than one week.

18. "Care over the barricade" refers to a situation in which a Paramedic passes instructions to third parties regarding how to provide medical care to patients that the Paramedic cannot access (i.e., hostages).

19. Concealment hides the Paramedic, whereas cover offers protection from gunfire. Concealment does not necessarily offer protection from gunfire.

20. To protect in place, the tactical medic must be provided cover, often associated with suppressive fire capability and armed protection, while care is being rendered.

Fill in the Blank

21. tactical medics

22. medical threat assessment

23. protect in place

24. suppressive fire, armed protection

25. concept of CAB